From Green Persimmons to Cranky Parrots

Practice management axioms to live by

From Green Persimmons to Cranky Parrots

Practice management axioms to live by

Written by:
Robert L. Slaton, Ed.D., FACMGA
Bob Manning
Clyde W. Jackson

Illustrations by:
Lyle Slaton

Published by:
Medical Group Management Association
104 Inverness Terrace East
Englewood, CO 80112
(303) 799-1111

Medical Group Management Association (MGMA) publications are intended to provide current and accurate information and are designed to assist MGMA members in becoming more familiar with the subject matter covered. Such publications are distributed with the understanding that MGMA does not render any legal, accounting or other professional advice. No representation or warranties are made concerning the application of legal or other principles discussed by the author(s) to any specific fact or situation, nor is any prediction made concerning how any particular judge, governmental official or other person will interpret or apply such principles. Specific factual situations should be discussed with professional advisors.

To Maureen, Mike, Danny, Tom, Lyle and Andrea.

To Eva, Bo, Rachel, Doc and Joseph.

To Michael.

TABLE of CONTENTS

FOREWORD

What we have here is a down-to-earth guide for practicing managers regardless of organizational rank. The authors' simple, direct suggestions about management practices belie the fact that their advice is well-grounded in both organizational theory and experience.

The "war stories" and anecdotes liberally sprinkled throughout contribute to the book's readability and practical usefulness. What is of particular value is that this book provides a reality test for the reader. If you haven't experienced many of the situations recounted so cleverly, you should quickly reconsider whether you are achieving a passing grade from the "School of Hard Knocks."

Another thing I appreciated about this book is that the authors freely admit that they don't have all the answers — that "all the pieces" in management don't fit together easily and comfortably. While we all know that as a dictum, some authors make it appear as if complex concerns can always be analyzed and resolved, Slaton, Manning and Jackson make it refreshingly clear that real world events set the stage for the play — and that those events often are not controllable.

The challenge for the reader and one I would highly recommend is not only to take the time to read this book from cover to cover but also to pause and reflect on the ten axioms — and then put your own twist on the topic. Management is a messy business and we each react according to our personal exposure to the depth of the swamp.

And this is what makes the book so valuable and yes, even fun. You know that everything isn't cast in concrete and can take time to test those axioms in the context of your personal base of experience.

One additional thing is certain about this book. The authors collectively must have enjoyed exchanging thoughts and bringing those infamous war stories into the context of their axioms. They also talk about how important it is to remember that managers can be paid to have fun. It struck me that our authors really enjoyed putting their thoughts down on paper.

Don't purchase this book if you are looking for that well-referenced academic approach, but by all means acquire it if you want to sample the authors' wisdom and are prepared to enjoy their free-flowing, no-guarantee advice about management.

Austin Ross, FACMGA
Vice President and
Executive Administrator Emeritus
Virginia Mason Medical Center
Seattle, Washington

T he authors are indebted to **Mike Slaton**, who read and re-read the entire manuscript, reacted to the ideas, renamed chapters and helped clarify the logic; **Bo Bourke** who critiqued the chapters as they were being developed and who offered unflagging moral support; **Mary G. Barry, M.D.**, for proofreading and technical advice; **David Wunderlin**, for proofreading; **Lynn Martin** for word processing support; and **Eric Wehder**, who gave technical assistance on the illustrations. Thanks to **Lyle Slaton**, not only for creating the paper clip character that appears on the cover and throughout the book, but also for the patience he demonstrated repeatedly as publication deadlines approached.

This book would not have been possible without the support of the Medical Group Management Association staff: **Fred E. Graham, II, Ph.D., FACMGA**, Senior Associate Executive Director, **Dennis L. Barnhardt, APR**, Director of Communications, **Barbara U. Hamilton, M.A.**, Library Resource Center Director, **Brenda E. Hull**, Communications Project Manager, **Stephanie S. Wyllyamz**, Communications Specialist, **Deborah V. Kennington**, Communications Administrative Secretary and **Martha Huckaby**, Administrative Assistant.

ACKNOWLEDGEMENTS

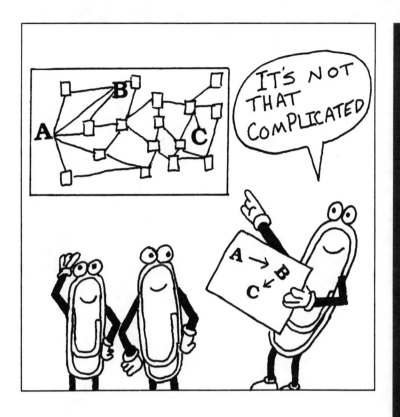

Folks, it's not that complicated

E ffective management rests on a few fundamental ideas. The trick is to understand them, take them to heart, and apply them consistently. "That's no way to build cars," was Detroit's response to a few simple ideas proposed by W. Edwards Deming after World War II. But in Japan he found an audience of car makers who understood his precepts. They took his rules to heart, applied them consistently, and had great success. Unfortunately, things got tough in Detroit and in the homes of American auto workers as a result.

New approaches to old ideas

In this book we list a few simple ideas about management. We call them axioms. You could call them techniques, approaches or methods, it doesn't matter. Call them "things to live by." The point is that these are fundamental ideas that work. In today's competitive times, applying these axioms can keep things from getting tough for you.

This book should be helpful at any point in your career, particularly if you have already read a dozen or two basic, classic or trendy books on management. Doing that will help put things in context. If you don't know the type of book we're talking about, find some bespectacled manager or executive and ask for the list. Like your authors, many managers have squandered their eyesight reading management books. With very little prompting we can all recite the litany of titles and authors' names. Just ask — we'll be flattered by your interest.

In addition to fitting in with the topical literature, this book fits into the real world. You will learn to recognize the real world after it has bitten you several times — that is, after you've had a few jobs managing people, made a lot of mistakes, gotten some more experience and made more mistakes. The way your own career began and developed will have an influence on how you read and use this book. What's here will make better sense to people whose careers began in the trenches, and who have made some real mistakes in their careers. In other words, this is not an academic treatise.

If you believe management is tidy and predictable (and especially if you've found a way to *make* it tidy and predictable), this book is not for you. We think management is fairly political. It hits you where you live. Management is about getting things done. We're not interested in how things are *supposed* to work; we're interested in how things *actually* work. Not only is management political, but it can get ugly. It makes babies cry and grown men weep. It's a furnace, a factory, a mill. Guess who's the grist? You are, if you're not careful.

So what are we trying to do with this book? We're just trying to keep you from getting all ground up. We're trying to save your hide. We think we can help you do a good job. It's more basic than that: we think we can help you *keep* your job, for heaven's sake. To some extent, the three managers who wrote this book have learned how to get things done. In the practical world, the ability to get things done is a valuable commodity. How to get things done is the focus of this book.

Do you remember the old story about the accountant who kept something locked in his desk, but would never tell anyone what it was? He would come to work each morning and look in the drawer, then relock it and go about his business. Finally one day he died, and his boss had to clean out the desk. Inside the drawer was a scrap of paper that had these words neatly printed on it: "Debits on the left, credits on the right." That's a good rule for getting things done if you are an accountant. It is something you should remember to say to yourself frequently. It's a rule you should always obey. (We recently heard that same old joke re-told, but this time it was about a surgeon instead of an accountant. The punch line was: "Spleen on the left, liver on the right.")

"Green side up!" is another of our favorite rules. It's a rule for getting things done if you are a sod layer. When you lay sod or when you supervise others who are laying sod, don't ever forget "Green side up."

To some degree, isn't that what management is all about — understanding and applying rules?

So, what rules do _managers_ have for getting things done? Well, we've listed some good ones in this book. These axioms are things you should understand, take to heart and apply consistently. They will save your hide.

Is there anything new in this book? Yes and no. Was there anything new about the pyramids? After all, aren't they just a bunch of old rocks? Well, maybe the arrangement was new — maybe the focus and placement was unusual.

So it is, perhaps, with this book. We have selected some good old stones, and stacked them up in a way that may be interesting and helpful to your development and survival as a manager.

Keeping it simple

Let's move to another topic. Here's a good line, uttered in exasperation by someone testifying at an investigation in Washington: "Senator, I guess I just can't make this _complicated enough_ for you to understand." Our approach to management is like that. We like to keep things simple. We're not saying management is easy — laying sod is not easy — we're just saying it doesn't have to be complicated.

Here is a slight diversion, to make a point:

In most businesses there is a small handful of things you can point to and say that the success of the business rests on them. You may have heard these referred to as "Critical Success Factors." For example, if you run a fruit stand, the products are perishable. For you, "inventory turnover" is a Critical Success Factor. You really have to keep tight control on inventory in your fruit business, because if the products spoil you can no longer sell them. You may do a fine job of selecting beautiful fruit, pricing it right, displaying it well, having helpful salespeople, keeping the floors clean, and so on, but if you let the fruit rot before the customers' eyes, your profits are going out with the garbage.

In every business it is important to identify the Critical Success Factors. There won't be many of them. While small in number, they are potent. By definition, no matter how good a job you do on the other aspects of your business, if you foul up even one of the Critical Success Factors, you're sunk. That's why they're called "critical." Physicians understand this concept immediately when you explain it in terms such as respiration and circulation. When those are present the patient has a chance. But if any one of the critical factors fails, the game is over.

What's the point? With management itself there is also a small handful of things you can point to and say, "If you do these, you'll stay in the game." We're going to tell you about those things in this book. They're really not all that complicated. They are axioms to live by.

In addition to the war stories, you will find lots of comparisons sprinkled throughout the book. Some of them are a bit overblown — like the one in the first chapter that says poor timing is like biting into a green persimmon. Or the one in the last chapter that says when you encounter problems it's like having a cranky parrot biting your finger. We don't apologize for the bold imagery. Our mission was to go from specific axioms to a general statement on management ... in other words, to boldly go where no one has gone before: from green persimmons to cranky parrots.

Now, it doesn't take much typesetting to list ten axioms. So where's the beef? What fills up the space between one axiom and the next? The meat of this book is in the case histories. We call them our "war stories" and we have lots of them to tell. We've included a fair number of them in this book to illustrate the axioms and to give you some clues to surviving your own wars. We didn't make up the war stories. They all happened to us or to people we know. Names and circumstances have been changed to avoid embarrassing ourselves more than absolutely necessary.

Now, let's deal with another issue: if you've read the table of contents, you might have concluded that *these "axioms" sound like clichés.* Ahem. Well, yes, they do. They are. That is, they *are* clichés — to people who have not been paying attention to the real world.

Someone famous said that every generation has the solemn obligation to repeat the obvious for the next generation. We believe that. Why? Because what's "obvious" to some must be discovered anew by others. We've learned through sad experiences to be grateful, not insulted, when someone takes the time to remind us of things we're already supposed to know.

What makes us think we're qualified to write this book? Well, it's not that we think we know everything about management. We don't know everything, but we do know a lot. We've fought a lot of battles, and we bear some wounds to prove it. We've won our share of those battles and we've learned a thing or two along the way. The three of us have management experience in an unusually wide variety of fields, including banking, retail, restaurant, government, the arts, information processing and, of course, medicine. Our experiences are helpful, but equally important is the perspective we have developed, which we have chosen as the editorial viewpoint for this book: we focus on the practical and we downplay what people *should* do so we can concentrate on what people *actually* do. We have distilled a lot of experience into ten axioms that, in our own lives, have allowed us to manage effectively in environments that on the surface had nothing in common.

So, we've been there. We're still there, and we're having the time of our lives.

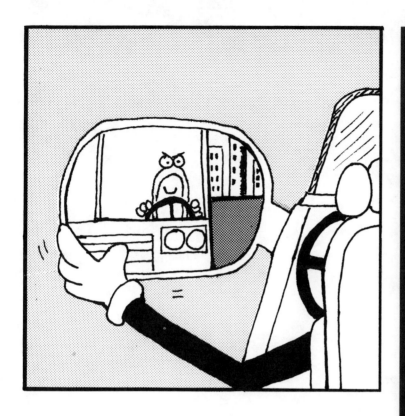

AXIOM

Timing is almost everything

1

A
nyone who drives a car can call to mind an example of
the axiom "Timing is almost everything." Just remember one of those times you almost got creamed on the
freeway entrance ramp. C'mon, you remember. It was
rush hour, and that guy in the blue minivan ... you
thought he was moving over to let you in, but he wasn't! So you
almost got mauled by that 18-wheeler, remember? It was scary.

Entering the expressway is easy — at 3 a.m., when there are no
other cars on the road. At other times, though, merging into traffic
can be challenging, unnerving, dangerous, even deadly. The same
holds true for lots of other things in life and in business: things are
easy when the timing is right, and difficult when it's not.

Some people are better than others at merging with fast-moving
traffic. Who are those people, and how did they get that way? We'd
say they are the people who have developed good timing. We'd say
timing is almost everything when it comes to getting on the freeway.

Let's continue this highway analogy and let's begin by dispelling
several myths.

Myth number one: *the kind-hearted motorist.* When you're
trying to get on the freeway, what are the chances that someone will
move over or slow down to let you in? After all, aren't there a lot of
kind-hearted and attentive drivers out there, people who will see the
value of letting you merge safely, even if it means adding a half-a-
second to their own journey?

Yes and no. Our scientific research indicates that people like that exist, *but there are none of them within 200 miles of you.* We can prove scientifically that where *you* are, nobody gives a hoot whether you get on the freeway or not.

Myth number two: *power and prestige are important.* Do people in big, fast, expensive new cars have an easier time merging into freeway traffic?

Are you kidding? They've got it worse than you do! In the battle for right-lane supremacy, position means power, and the accelerator is the great equalizer.

The right lane of the interstate is a fertile breeding ground for contempt. In the anonymity of traffic, all those ugly urges we normally suppress are free to burst forth. And they do. With vigor. Burdened with our burdens, what do we do when we see a carefree, new, red, $60,000 two-seater with the top down, trying to merge ahead of us? Do we slow down and let 'em in?

Ha! What we do is ... Well, it's just *too* vile, isn't it?

Myth number three: *a smile and a wave will sometimes get you in.* This is not a myth. This is the truth.

The point is that things on the freeway aren't all that different from things in your office:

- You're on your own, and nobody else is all that interested in what you're trying to do; although
- Some people are benignly indifferent; and
- A few people are actively hostile.

Timing: a key to success

We're going to show that timing is crucial to getting things done, and to converting indifference and hostility to support. We will start with an Abraham Lincoln story and a sports analogy — the only sports analogy in the whole book. Then we'll discuss the fact that timing always points to something else; we'll give examples of how to affect timing; and we'll touch briefly on the relationship between timing and power.

The literature on management contains a great deal of discussion about timing. Some say "timing is everything." We say timing is a*lmost* everything. By "timing" we simply mean knowing when to act, and when not to act; when to make a move, and when to sit still; when to initiate change, and when to maintain the status quo; when to approach the boss with a problem or a new idea, and when to stay the heck down at your end of the hall.

Military history is full of stories of successes and failures based on timing. The Civil War has many examples showing how defeat befell brigades or divisions that simply moved too early or too late.

Political history, too, teaches the same lesson. Successful politicians are almost always masters of timing. Among the foremost was Abraham Lincoln, who wrote the Emancipation Proclamation months before it was issued — and then simply put it in his desk. He knew the timing was not right. At the time Lincoln wrote the Proclamation, Union armies had suffered a series of defeats; Lincoln knew the Proclamation would be viewed as a desperate act by a government about to fail. Periodically he would take the document out of his desk and make revisions. He waited until the Union armies were winning, and then issued the Proclamation from a position of strength. He waited until the time was right!

Now for the obligatory sports analogy. A vivid example of the value of timing comes from an "offside" error in pro football.

If you don't know the game, here's what happens: the two teams are lined up, ready for the next play to begin. The very biggest members of one team (the team's "front line") will be lined up side-by-side, facing the other team's front line, one-against-one, with the football resting on the ground between the two lines. The play begins when the ball is lifted off the ground by one of the players. This happens quite suddenly. But until the ball is moved, none of the normal rowdiness is allowed.

Sometimes a player will get rowdy before the ball is lifted, and he'll go charging forward into the opposing line. This is called an "offside" violation. When it happens the referees get excited. They throw little yellow flags around, and blow their whistles and wave their arms. But most important of all, they penalize the offending team for their rowdy behavior.

Wait a minute. When players get rowdy, aren't they just doing what everyone expects of football players? *Yes!* It's what the coaches tell the players to do. It's what the opposing players and referees anticipate happening. It's what the fans pay their money to see. So what's the difference between "offside" rowdiness and regular rowdiness? The only difference is timing. In one instant, in one blink of an eye, the behavior changes from being inappropriate (even a violation of the rules) to being expected, anticipated, desired.

Whew! *That* is the difference timing can make.

The reality of timing

Is timing like rhythm — you're either born with it or you're not? Luckily, no. Some people do seem to have a knack for it, but all managers can improve their timing.

How? Just remember how you learned to cross the street safely. What were you told? That's right: "Stop, look, and listen!" You weren't told, "Run like heck and hope no cars are coming!" Crossing the street isn't about speed and agility — it is about timing.

"Stop, look, and listen!" is advice for improving your timing, and it works as well in the complicated area of medical management as it does on your Sunday stroll. The simple technique of *stopping before you act to consider consequences and alternatives* will help you improve timing.

Timing, more than anything else, is the art of anticipating — anticipating a need or opportunity, objections, responses, proposals, counter-proposals, counter-responses. Nobody can see the future, but with practice most people can make educated guesses.

Timing always points to something else

Timing always points to something else. First and foremost, timing points to the fact that all actions involving more than one person succeed or fail on the basis of politics — the interplay of individuals to achieve desired ends.

In any group action, all the members of the group have their own individual (and seldom completely harmonious) agendas. Achieving success requires satisfying everyone's wishes, or at the very least, convincingly demonstrating that the proposed action will not interfere with anyone's wishes. Some people know their real agendas, and state them openly. As one physician said in response to a proposal, "I don't care what you do about that, but don't you dare diddle with my dough."

Others do not always state their agendas openly. They may be suspicious of any action whatever, because they have not studied their own position carefully. We all know people who resist every idea that is not their own. We all know people who insist money is not the issue — and yet take you to the wall over every cent.

Self interest is the engine that propels most human activity. Whenever you propose to do something involving others, you engender a healthy skepticism in them as they warily evaluate your proposal against their own self interest. This happens unfailingly, every time action is proposed. People do things for *their* reasons, not yours, and they do things *their* ways, not yours. It is pointless to hope your clear logic will eliminate this response. It won't. Logic is not the foundation of most business decisions anyway. Your only shot at gaining cooperation from others is to present your proposals in terms of *their* reasons for cooperating with them.

For every purpose you state in a proposal, someone else might easily have an opposite purpose with equal validity. (The validity arises from the politics, not the logic.) Opposition frequently hinges on money, priorities, personnel, procedures or any other item from the laundry list of reasons for not doing what's been proposed, or for not doing it now. These reasons may be legitimate, but they rarely tell the whole story.

You know those candies that melt in your mouth, not in your hand? Agenda items are like those candies. Both have a brightly colored outside shell, and something altogether different in the center. You can't separate the two parts. You're supposed to chew 'em up together. The outer surface of an agenda item is the claimed or purported reason the item exists. The inside is the political core. You have to take both flavors together, even if you really only have a taste for one of them.

In other words, if your timing recognizes only the visible aspect of the agenda item, and ignores the political element, you're probably in trouble.

Most people have found themselves in this situation: someone does not want to do something you proposed; you have good reasons for your proposal — it's the right thing, it will save money, and so on. You try to deal with the opposition rationally and sensitively. You go to great trouble to be diplomatic. Yet you manage to arouse open anger and determined, public resistance from that person.

You haven't just entered the Twilight Zone; you've just bumped into a hidden agenda item. If you persist in dealing with the stated reasons, you run the risk of unmasking the person. Unmasking others by successfully rebutting their stated reasons for opposing an action can be very dangerous, because it can expose the political core of their opposition.

As managers we must time proposals and actions for those magic moments when people are receptive and the environment is right. If we do a good job politically, everything else is a cakewalk. The actions we suggest will seem eminently sensible; they will appear to be foregone conclusions; and they will seem to have come from the mind of the group as a whole, instead of from our own mischievous, fertile little brains.

Come to think of it, the heart of successful management is finding reasons for people with different agendas and motivations to cooperate on the same issue. Remember the challenge of merging onto an expressway: Try to force your left front fender into an opening and you evoke resistance and retaliation. But smile, wave — do what it takes to get cooperation — and you slip right in. Our own behavior, then, can influence timing.

How to affect timing

One of the enduring cultural legends of the American West is that of the Rainmaker. The Rainmaker's job, if you think about it, was nothing but an exercise in timing. If the Rainmaker could just manage to arrive at parched little towns two or three days ahead of the rain, he could drum up some business. Arriving one day late was equivalent to suicide.

We doubt that Rainmakers could really change the weather; the lucky ones simply took advantage of timing. But in business there actually are ways you can change "atmospheric conditions" that accompany your proposals. Here are some tried and proven methods:

Wait until there is enough pain that your proposal will be welcome.

To do this you may even have to endure some discomfort yourself, but at least you'll know there's a happy ending in store for everyone.

Here's a good tip: A few well-thought-out questions can make people anticipate pain, and reduce your waiting time. For example: "I'm not really sure how the new reporting requirements affect us. Does anyone have any ideas of how the physicians will have to comply?" You may know exactly how it affects physicians. You may know exactly how it affects medical records and other operations.

The response you want is: "What requirement? Does it mean *I* have to do something?" You then have the opening to say, "Let me look at it and summarize what it seems to say, and let's talk about it. I'm not really sure how big this monster is, but we can probably get it in a cage."

Pain hurts. Anticipatory pain gives you an opportunity to help avoid the real pain.

Make plans before you need them.

Don't bother talking seriously to superiors about an issue that is not of current concern. Follow Lincoln's example: prepare a plan and keep it in drawer until the timing is right.

In one situation, a clinic administrator talked for months about starting an occupational medicine program, but the clinic leaders were not receptive. When a local manufacturing plant waved money and asked for help in handling workers compensation cases, those same clinic leaders wanted a plan "right now." Their response was a typical, and valid, boss's response — "Take the money ... we can work out the details later." The clinic administrator had developed a plan in the meantime and it was ready to execute. He delivered the occupational medicine program "right now" with a minimum of disruption. Everybody won, and the boss was impressed.

A good administrator anticipates needs and opportunities, and then draws up plans — to various states of completion. The administrator might ultimately propose the plans, or might continue to develop them, or may eventually discard them, all depending on need and the politics of timing.

Some plans will never see the light of day. This is normal. But be hard-nosed in reviewing your performance. If very few of your plans ever go anywhere, you must seriously ask if you really understand the fundamental propositions of your business, and the political realities of your organization.

Get a lightning rod — hire a consultant.

One of the best functions of a consultant is to give bad news, and then go away. Some people resist change so much that they must have a scapegoat. Skilled consultants understand this need, and can focus the issues clearly, and serve as a lightning rod for all of the negative feelings. When this happens, the human urge to kill the messenger is directed toward someone outside the organization, leaving you free to form partnerships and address the issues.

It is important to understand the role of consultants. They are not supposed to tell you how to run your organization; instead, they are to be a resource to help you run it. A skilled consultant will not tell you what to do or take an operational role, even when you insist on it.

Here's an oft-repeated scenario:

A consultant reviewed operations and wrote a candid report. It said that there were major problems with the organization, that the senior leaders were not in agreement about objectives, that various systems for accomplishing work were ineffective and that the political battles among the senior staff seriously limited the potential of the organization. The report then said that all these problems could be fixed through effective senior management. It said someone needed to start laying down guidelines and holding people accountable. The problem was a perceived vacuum of leadership at the top.

The consultant was paid well for the report, although no one liked it. Most were angry at it. But economic realities made them deal with the issues, and the consultant had in fact identified the root of the dysfunction. Eventually this knowledge turned into power, which was applied toward action. Things improved.

The humorist Garrison Keillor says that telling people a truth they have successfully avoided for years "is not a pretty thing." Hire a consultant to do ugly chores like that.

Listen to the needs of others.

Really listen. Really, truly, *be-quiet-and-listen* listen. Your own employees can often tell you what's wrong, can often tell you how to fix it and can often tell you when the time is right for action.

Listening to others helps you understand their needs, and helps you design the tools, methods and systems that will fill those needs. You won't have to force anyone to use a tool that they perceive they had a hand in designing. Those people will hound *you* (instead of the other way around), wondering why it's taking you so long to implement "their" ideas.

Another benefit of listening is that you will often find additional reasons to do what you wanted to do anyway. This leads us to the next way to affect timing.

Never do anything for just one reason.

That's being smart, not devious. Most organizations (like most people) have finite resources — and unlimited desires. It's smart to think through the number of needs you can satisfy with available resources and with one proposal. As we used to say down on the farm, "If the truck is going to town anyway, let's haul everything we can, both ways, on the trip."

Patient flow is always a hot topic, so let's use it as an example. Let's suppose you've listened carefully to what everyone has to say on the topic. (An aside: don't forget to listen to *patients* when you're talking about patient flow.) And then you carefully diagrammed and documented the problem and some proposed solutions. Great work, all done in the name of "finding ways to keep physicians from having to wait for charts and patients." Who wouldn't support that?

The result of all your legwork, brainwork and flow-charting will (we trust) be an improvement in the flow of patients through the office. But coincidentally, didn't you also just give yourself the information you need to justify the cost of the clinic management software you've wanted for two years? After all, if you can demonstrate increased income from seeing two or three more patients per day, it's a "no-brainer" to pay for the software.

Will the upgraded clinic management software interface better with the word processing and medical transcription software? It may, or it may not. The point is to consider all the loads that need to be hauled, both ways, on the trip.

11

The beautifully-detailed notes you kept while solving this problem might make an interesting case study for others to read. Isn't that a requirement for becoming a Fellow in the American College of Medical Group Administrators? Do tell. You have saved it in a word processor for future reference, haven't you? Good. You can use it to illustrate a point in a book, an article or a speech.

You see the point. Make it part of your management discipline when proposing action to identify as many valid reasons as possible. As long as the truck makes the trip ...

Repackage your idea.

No one wants to install a computer system just for the sake of having a computer system. But everyone wants to improve patient services and to improve earnings. People will gladly install a computer system, or comply with new regulations, or do a lot of other things in order to take care of patients and make more money. Repackaging the idea in politically acceptable terms affects the timing.

Never force an idea before its time.

Persimmons. Strange fruit from a scrawny tree, but with a good taste. Just don't try to eat one before the first frost. It may look ready, but it's not. The experience of biting into a persimmon before its time is both indescribable and unforgettable. Your mouth puckers down to the size of a skin pore, and becomes so parched you'll think all the water in the world will not relieve the dryness — all this while you're enduring a taste somewhat like a combination of green tomatoes, overripe bananas and rotten apples. The good news is that you cannot eat enough of them to make you sick.

On the other hand, you *can* force an idea before its time, and that can make you and others sick. It can even destroy your career. When you think you understand the political timing and think you have stated your ideas in terms that match the needs of the group, don't charge ahead. Stop, look, and listen. Make sure you're not about to chomp a green persimmon. Verify everything with everyone who will be affected. Ask each person: "Do you see any other issues we should address before going forward? Are we ready to go ahead?" It is fun to have the timing right, and to feel certain you're right before you charge ahead.

If at first you don't succeed, don't pout.

Pouting casts a pall over everything, including the other projects you're trying to accomplish — you know, the ones there's still some hope for. Pouting publicly is like putting a sign saying "Pull me!" on a chain around your neck. Pouting makes your emotions the focus of disrespect instead of making your competence an issue of respect.

Here's a good rule about selling: If you talk to the right people at the right times about the right things in the right way, you will make sales. If you do not make sales, one or more of those things is not right. If you were unable to sell your idea, one of those things is not right. Don't pout — get busy.

Now that we have mentioned some techniques for affecting timing, let's get back to one of the core truths of management. Like management itself, timing involves power, and hinges on how you understand and relate to power, how you use and share power.

Timing and power

Managers like to control things: people, processes, agendas, events. That's one of the characteristics that makes people want to become managers. But in the absence of discipline, that trait can turn people into bad managers. In order to develop good timing you will have to learn how to share power while retaining power. This topic is discussed at length in another chapter, but here are some quick tips:

- The issues the boss perceives as important, are;

- The boss's time is more important than yours;

- Your peers' perception of your use of power can destroy your project, regardless of your timing. Great timing cannot overcome brute strength; and

- Like you, your employees also want to control their own pace and timing, their own time and environment. If you are smart you will help them do it.

Final thoughts

A good bit of the discussion about timing in this chapter has focused on being patient, being able to wait. But in the final analysis, timing must be directed toward getting something *done.* Delays and postponements are often a part of the process, but let's not lose sight of the goal. Waiting is always done in anticipation of something. Timing implies movement. "Stop, look, and listen" is not an end in itself; you're not standing on the corner because you want to spend your time stopping, looking, and listening. You're there to get across the street. "Stop, look, and listen" is the means for getting something done. At some point you've got to act. Do something. *Get the lead out.*

Back to the entrance ramp of the expressway. Of all the drivers you encounter trying to get on the freeway, who do you hate the most? Our vote goes to those who *stop* at the end of the ramp before entering the freeway.

Here's you, craning your neck to the left as you glide down the ramp, looking out your side window and checking your side mirror, praying for one small bit of daylight between cars. You're ready to floor it! You take one last, quick glance up front ... and you nearly plow into the car ahead, because the driver ahead *stopped dead*, waiting for the next big break in traffic. Which, on this particular road, won't occur until 3 a.m. On Sunday. The 16th of March. In the year 2008.

On the expressway and in your business, pay attention to timing, so someone doesn't run up against your rear end.

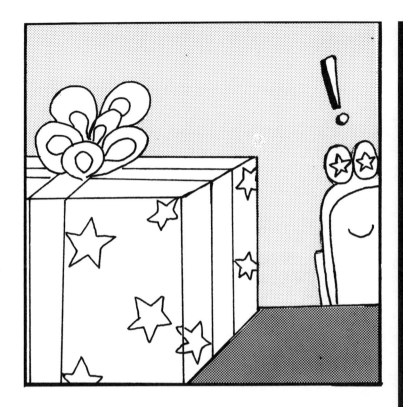

Packaging
is
everything
that timing
is not

AXIOM 2

W e know an office where the annual holiday gift exchange is enhanced by this unusual twist: Each person's name is put in a hat three times. Here's how this works. Each person brings a gift (just one gift) and places it on a table. Then they draw names, one at a time. The first person takes a gift from the table. The second person takes a package from the table or the package selected by the first person. From then on, when your name is called, you get to decide whether to take a gift from the table or from someone else (and no fair picking the package you brought.)

After a while the table is empty, and everyone has a package. But remember, each person's name is going to come up three times before the drawing is over. So once the table is empty, when your name is called again, you must either keep the present you have, or exchange it with someone else. ("Exchange" is a polite word for "grab what they have and make them take the one you didn't want.")

Everyone has a ball trying to determine the desirability of the gifts on the basis of the packaging — and on the basis of how much someone else seems to want to hang on to what they have. And unlike most selection processes, where the first person to choose always has the best selection, here the *last* person called gets the best choice — because nobody can take that gift away. This means the strategy for getting the package you want is not to pick it right away, and (once you get your hands on the one you really want) to pretend it's *not* the one you want, in order to discourage others from taking it away.

The crowning irony, of course, is that for all their caginess, nobody knows what's inside the packages they're selecting. Everyone might as well be blindfolded. The worst looking package might contain the nicest gift, while the best looking package might be nothing but window dressing for a decidedly mediocre gift.

But the participants must base their evaluations on something, and because there's not much to go on, appearance rules the day. After the final selection, everyone opens the gifts at once. Naturally, some people nod smugly when the contents are in fact appropriate to the wrapping; others scream in laughter when the packaging was clearly, misleadingly (and often intentionally) inappropriate.

Packaging gets attention

This chapter is about packaging. That is a topic that can cover a great deal of territory, beginning with the way you present your practice to your patients, all the way to the how you deliver good news and bad news to your staff. In this chapter we will focus on one main aspect — the way you package and deliver your ideas and proposals. But you can apply the principles to any type of packaging.

Presenting your ideas is not like attending the party described above. The object of the party is to yuk it up, sometimes at the small expense of yourself and others. But the object of presenting your ideas is to have them accepted — to get approval of your plans and commitment to your projects. Presuming your ideas are reasonable, then *knowing when and how to present them* is all there is to getting them accepted. Really.

Knowing when to present ideas was discussed in the last chapter.

How to present your ideas is the topic of this chapter. If you do a good job on both these things, *success is a foregone conclusion.* This is utterly true, and can't be said more simply than that. That's the whole shootin' match, the whole ball of wax. That's all there is. Timing and packaging. One, two. Timing is nearly everything; packaging is everything that timing is not.

Said another way: *Nothing will sink a proposal faster than sloppy packaging.*

One of the authors of this book, early in his career, was asked on short notice to write and present a report analyzing the changes needed in a program run by a state agency. It took three weeks of using a friend's apartment 10 hours a day to gather and analyze the material, to develop and test recommendations and to write the report.

The content of the report was excellent. But the agency director rejected the report with only a cursory glance at the first page. The typos and strike-overs screamed out "carelessness." There was no cover page or binding. The report looked bad.

"Aw, give the kid a break," you say; "The deadline was impossible and there was way too much material to cover, and still he got it done." Sorry. No one was interested in that. The poor packaging kept the report from being considered by the director, which meant that the people who really needed to see it would not see it. Not only were three weeks wasted, but analyses and recommendations that might benefit a lot of people would not be acted upon.

So the report (and by extension its author) was unfairly branded "careless." That's bad, but it could have been worse: it could have been "laughable."

Most of us have a primal fear of being laughed at. Good. That fear serves us well in our careers. Few experiences can devastate your standing and your self-image the way having a group laugh at your presentation can. This is truly something to worry about.

Come on now, people don't really laugh at each other do they? Of course not ... and the tooth fairy will come tonight, just after the Easter Bunny leaves, right before your ship comes in. Granted, outright laughter in a business setting is unusual and an extreme reaction. But it can happen. And, because it indicates a fundamental and untreatable lack of respect, it is always fatal to the presentation.

Wait a minute. Won't good ideas stand on their own? Of course they will. Right after ... well, you know the rest of the sentence. Unlike the fun at the end of the Christmas party, in a business presentation, if the package looks bad, no one will open it to see what's inside.

That's the bad news. The good news is that you have complete control over the packaging. You control the ribbon, the wrapping paper, the box and what's in it; you control everything. You can dress up your ideas any way you please.

And you *should* dress them up. They deserve it, don't they? You worked hard on them, didn't you?

Hmmm. Well, now. Apparently we're going to have to be stern with you. Remember, this is for your own good. Here it is: If you don't care enough about your ideas to package them attractively, maybe you deserve the lack of consideration you undoubtedly receive.

Sorry to be so blunt, but trust us: there are much worse ways to learn that lesson than reading it in a book. Now, let's talk about some of these elements of packaging you control.

You are the ribbon

Guess what? You are part of the package. In the long ago, before cellophane tape was invented, ribbons had a practical function: they tied up packages. They kept wrapping paper in place and kept box lids from coming open. In the long, *long ago*, before ribbon itself was invented, some other functional-but-dull material like twine, rope or rawhide would have served those important purposes.

But nowadays, a ribbon's purpose is purely psychological. It is there to announce that something special is in your midst, something valuable and desirable.

A well-selected and carefully-tied ribbon entices people to action. Polite people untie ribbons; the rest of us just rip them to shreds trying to get to the goodies. In either event the psychological function has been served.

When you make a business presentation you are the ribbon. The way others perceive you determines whether they'll select your package or move on to another. Your dress, grooming, vocabulary, demeanor, interaction skills and other observable characteristics will create a bias in the people you encounter. Almost automatically, their reaction to your ideas will begin leaning in the same direction.

If you don't try to impress people favorably, you'll get just what you tried for: They'll probably ignore you and your ideas. And if something about you actually annoys them, your ideas certainly won't get a full hearing.

But on the other hand, if something about you strikes them favorably — your professionalism, the depth of your knowledge of the subject, your thorough understanding of not only the issues and the consequences, but also the often-overlooked opportunities — whatever it is, your ideas are getting a boost because you've taken the time to package them properly. Give as much attention to marketing yourself as you give to developing those ideas.

You may want to look at some "_(Blank)_ for Success" books. You can fill in the blank with words such as dress, negotiate or speak; it is easy to find books on the topic. Another approach is to ask a trusted and competent friend — someone outside your organization — for feedback on the image you present. But remember this proverb: "Be careful what you wish for, because you might get it!" Make sure you really want the feedback, and that you are prepared for whatever you might hear. Have you ever misunderstood the request for honest feedback? You thought the former friend meant it, didn't you?

You may also want to spend some time with a reputable career counselor or consultant, even a clinical psychologist, to discuss how you present yourself. But don't bother talking about this at home, where people like you too much to be honest, or they're _too_ honest, or they don't know what they're talking about, or they _do_ know what they're talking about, but you don't believe them. At least those are the possibilities at our homes.

Because you are part of the packaged proposal, it will be identified with you; the way people react to you will influence how they feel about the proposal. **Caution:** don't become so identified with the proposal that if it is rejected, you are rejected. That is a danger with projects you feel strongly about, like those that just took three weeks of 10-hour days. It is good that you worked on the proposal as though your life depended on it, but you have to be able to abandon ship if it runs aground.

It is important to do good work, and to take pride in your work. Still, you don't have to stake your reputation on everything you do. Some things are more important than others. Some projects will be exciting for you, and some will be dull. Regardless, do remember that your own feelings will color others' perceptions. Your own feelings are like the color and the sheen of the ribbon. Others will begin to evaluate the contents of the package before it is even opened, based on how you feel about it yourself.

A quick summary is the wrapping paper

In mystery novels everything is explained on the last page. In business writing it's just the opposite: everything is explained on the first page. Introduce *every* presentation with a summary, whether the presentation is written or oral, long or short, simple or complex, board room formal or lunch room casual. Make the summary attractive. Wrap your proposal in it. Use it to make your audience want to see and hear more.

How long does it take to read a one-page summary? A couple of minutes at most. That's how long you have to get people interested in your proposal. The scope of the project doesn't matter — you can be asking to upgrade the phone system, or you can be proposing to make war on the entire galaxy, it doesn't matter: you've got two minutes to summarize your case.

Your summary should give people an incentive to continue listening, to delve further. It should serve the same function as attractive wrapping paper on a package: it should make the recipient want to tear through it quickly to get to the goodies.

Your summary will undoubtedly be interesting — *to you.* In the previous chapter we mentioned that people tend to do things for their own reasons, not yours. Call that to mind when you are preparing your summary, and make a conscious effort to address the self-interest of the people in your audience. Answer the following questions: Why should this audience listen to me for even two minutes? Why should they listen to me after two minutes? Have I really done my homework? Do I have a written proposal ready? Do I have backup data? Is my presentation clear?

A technique the authors use is asking our listeners for two minutes of their time, saying that at the end of the two minutes we will leave or continue, their decision. At the beginning of the presentation we hand a watch to someone to call time. Ninety seconds or so later, we ask if they want to continue. You had better believe that we get our packaging together before going into that presentation. We even practice our presentations with a tape recorder or a video camera, replaying the tapes to critique ourselves. Try this yourself. It can be helpful — and humbling.

The "give me two minutes" technique does not work well with every audience, and in fact we don't actually use it very often — we simply prepare every presentation as though we were using it. It seems to help focus our thinking, reminding us that audiences need constant incentives to continue to pay attention. Appeal to your audience's self-interest, and in the first few minutes nail down the reasons they should hear out the rest of your presentation.

In written reports of course you don't have a chance to hand someone a watch. Don't worry; all readers come equipped with mental watches. Readers will time you without being asked.

In written reports you must grab the reader's attention quickly, just as you would if you were there in person. The same principle applies. The first few minutes are the wrapping paper on the package. In that time you must entice people to stay with you for the duration, to stick around and see what is inside.

An outline of "benefits and trade-offs" is the box

How much fun would it be to sit and open presents that weren't for you? Not much; the purpose (and the thrill) of ripping open a present is to get a quick and definite answer to one of life's simple, fundamental and ever-present questions: "What's in it for me?"

The next layer of packaging, and the next part of your presentation, must address that question head on. Don't leave this part out, and don't leave it up to the audience's imagination. Tell them straight out what's in it for them.

Your proposal won't float without support, and it will sink completely if it is actively opposed by those who wield the power to make the decisions. You must do all you can to gain support and to neutralize opposition. Now, you know the political environment of your own organization better than we do, but let us recommend a novel approach: tell the truth, the whole truth and nothing but the truth. Blurt it out: "I think this remodeling will help the Lab; it will help X-ray; it won't help Medical Records, but it won't hurt them either; and as far as Bookkeeping goes, it will make things even more uncomfortable until we can fix their problems next year."

Try to see your proposal from the perspective of each person affected, and then honestly lay out the resulting benefits, costs and trade-offs they will experience. Show them the rewards they will receive for their support (or non-opposition). Put your best foot forward, of course, but put all the cards on the table.

The project itself is what's inside the packaging

When you clean up after a party, what gets thrown away? The ribbons, the wrapping paper, the boxes ... all that pretty packaging that people worked on so hard. Everybody took the gifts with them, and they pitched the packaging. Oh, well.

Packaging is very important, but don't forget that it serves a temporary purpose. Everyone expects there to be something more permanent, and of more substantial value, inside that pretty package. After all, the package is just packaging.

In the central part of your presentation you will cover the details of what you are proposing to do. Then you'll recap everything you've said. These elements are critical, of course. But (again presuming your idea is a good one) if you've done a good job on the summary and the cost/benefit outline, these parts of the presentation are just a necessary formality. The hard part — the part where you actually sell your idea — will already be over.

Let's have a short war story about a talented and ambitious mid-level administrator at a clinic we know. The story turns on an issue of timing, but it also has a "good things come in small packages" aspect to it. You'll see the small package in the part of the story where the administrator delivers — get this — a one-sentence summary and a one-sentence cost/benefit outline. See if you can find where this lovely, small bit of packaging is hidden in the story.

Her name was Isabella Consuella Moore, but everyone called her "I.C." She was ambitious, as we said, and she had an eye toward expanding her responsibilities by creating a marketing department. She tried floating the idea a few times, but nobody else was terribly interested.

Then, as a result of some mixed signals during a reorganization, one of the most-high senior administrators ended up being moved to an office that was not appropriate to his position in the organization. He was really, um, displeased at this turn of events, and let everyone know it. Constantly. "I am really displeased at this turn of events," he would say, or words to that effect.

Like a hangnail, this was starting to require a disproportionate amount of attention. And it was obvious the problem wasn't about to go away without some action. This was becoming a big, ugly, hairy gorilla of a problem.

Now, in addition to a good mind, I.C. had a great office. She started looking around. Near the main administration area she found a large section of converted exam rooms that weren't being put to very good use. It wasn't a particularly nice section, but it would serve her purposes.

I.C. hinted to another of the most-high senior administrators that if the clinic ever did decide to create a marketing department, I.C. knew where it could go: down there in those converted exam rooms. And, she supposed, if she was in charge of the department, she'd probably have to go down there, too — even if it meant giving up her nice office — which the unhappy administrator coveted.

(Did you just miss the small package?)

Needless to say, eyes opened wide, smiles spread across faces, and people who had been unenthusiastic were now staunch supporters of creating a marketing department. Of course they didn't just say "Go do it." This was a well-run clinic, and so there were lots of questions to answer, lots of hoops to jump through. But I.C. had anticipated all that, and had diagrams, flow-charts, budgets and analyses ready. Within a matter of days she and the three new, hand-picked staff members moved to the new location. Everybody won.

Related thought

Here's a related thought, not about packaging but still important and relevant. You will undoubtedly have to make promises to get support for your ideas. (I.C., for example, had to promise that the Marketing Department would more than pay for itself in increased revenue for the clinic.) *What you promise, deliver.* Can it be said more simply than that?

In fact, you'll do well to under-promise and over-deliver. But at the very least, do what you said you'd do.

Now back to the main topic. In this chapter we made an analogy between a nicely-wrapped gift and a formal business presentation. We also showed how I.C. Moore managed to wrap up one idea in just two sentences — admittedly in perfect circumstances. (Remember, timing is nearly everything.) Ideas can be packaged in a variety of ways. Some of those ways are not pleasant. Sometimes you feel like an idea has just been delivered to you in the nose cone of a Scud missile. And sometimes you might reciprocate in the same way. The point is that it's important to assess your audience, and to package your ideas and your messages in an appropriate manner.

One of the authors once worked in a place where he wrote a series of memos on a variety of topics. His boss called him in one day, read one of the memos aloud, discussed it with him, and then tore up the memo. The process was repeated for 30 or 40 minutes. It became very clear that the boss didn't want memos, he wanted discussion. The tradition in that organization was oral. It was something every newcomer had to learn. It wasn't written down anywhere. (Naturally.) Again, the point is to package your ideas appropriately.

Now, to clarify another issue. Remember when we talked about the poor packaging that scuttled the report for the state agency? Did you notice we didn't blame a "lack of packaging" for the bad result? That is a point worth mentioning. There's no such thing as lack of packaging; there's only a lack of good or adequate packaging. You can't *not* package your ideas. You can try, but remember it's the recipient (not you) who perceives and judges the packaging. If you try to ignore the packaging, the recipients won't conclude that your packaging is non-existent; they'll merely decide your packaging is bad. You simply have no choice about controlling the packaging. It is like the silly, true statement, "Everybody has to be somewhere."

Final thoughts

An investor purchased 1,000 shares of an obscure over-the-counter stock from a broker. The next week the stock went up three points. The investor bought another 1,000 shares. The stock again rose three points. Then the investor bought 5,000 shares. The stock rose eight points. Smelling a profit, the investor told the broker to sell all the stock. The broker asked, "To whom?" The investor had been the only purchaser.

Misleading packaging can be like that. It can bedazzle. It can be the wool that gets pulled over someone's eyes. But people don't stay dazzled and misled for long. Chickens come home to roost. Give your great ideas a great presentation. But don't let any half-baked ideas out of the oven until they're done. Most ideas have to incubate for a while. Think of them as a birthday cake you're making for a friend; all your careful measuring and mixing will be a goopy mess if you don't leave it in the oven long enough. Make sure it's done. Only then do you get to bring it out, decorate it and put on the candles. Then, light that sucker up, and sing for all you're worth!

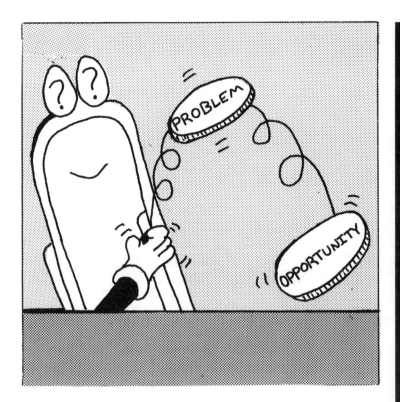

You never have a problem — only an opportunity

I n this chapter, we will make the point that problems and opportunities are the flip sides of the same coin — you can't have one without the other. Every person and every business has a collection of these coins and they must choose which side of the coins they're going to display to the world.

In this chapter we will also show that you can give your career a push if, instead of hiding from problems, you actively look for them.

We will cover some interesting ground — from a schoolhouse in the country to a university medical center in the big city, with stops in between. Along the way we'll throw in some war stories and some business tips. At the journey's end, we hope you will have arrived at a conclusion: "You never have a problem — only an opportunity."

Perception determines treatment

Let's begin with a story many people may have heard:

A young farm boy came home from school with this note pinned to his coat: "Dear Parents — Your son Jonathan comes to school wearing soiled clothes. Sometimes his face is dirty and he smells. Signed, Teacher."

Jonathan's father, a hard-working farmer who needed the boy's help before school, replied: "Dear Teacher — Johnny's a farm boy, not a rose. I send him to school to get smart, not smelt. Signed, Johnny's father."

31

The farmer may have understood a principle that the teacher didn't: how you *perceive* a thing will often set the pattern for how you *treat* that thing. Your preconceptions can sometimes exert more of an influence on you than the objective evidence does.

The teacher thought of Jonathan as a student. Students are supposed to look, act and smell a certain way. Jonathan didn't fit the mold; he was a problem that required fixing. But the father thought of Jonathan as a farm boy who was lucky enough to be enrolled in school. As far as the father was concerned the boy fit the mold just fine, thank you.

Thomas Cummings makes the same point in his book, *Systems Theory for Organizational Development.* He speaks of the person who searches for the truth by turning over a thousand rocks and looking under them. Then he says, "The angle of the view may be more important than what is under the rock."

Our third axiom is, "You never have a problem — only an opportunity." We've heard this repeated so often (and so often inappropriately) we've wanted to gag. But in fact this one is the most important of our axioms. This one is the "biggie." What you believe about this axiom will have profound consequences on your career.

Perception determines outcome

Let's use the beginning of a war story to illustrate what we mean. The situation: The clinic administrator rounded the corner to the main hallway one morning and walked squarely into Dr. Godley at the peak of a Force Ten Tantrum. Other people were spinning on their heels to get out of the way. Registration clerks and medical assistants cowered like puppies as the doctor continued his outburst. Spying the administrator, the doctor turned his rage upon him. "You there!" he bellowed in his very loudest you-better-snap-to-attention voice. "Why can't we do this one simple thing: why can't we get the doctor, the patient and the medical record in the same room at the same time?"

Have you faced a situation like that in your career? Was it a problem ... or an opportunity? How you perceived the situation probably determined the outcome.

If you view the above incident as a problem, something sneaky happens: the problem multiplies. You have not one, but many, problems. Just to list a few: an unhappy doctor, unhappy employees, an embarrassed administrator, a turf war, a desire to teach the doctor he can't treat people like that, and so on.

Luckily, our administrator had the good sense to view this as an opportunity — an unusually good opportunity, in fact, because Dr. Godley had done all the groundwork.

Most people that day were saying Dr. Godley had put everyone in an uproar. They said he had angered, frightened or alienated the staff, had read the riot act, had barked out marching orders, had threatened that heads would roll.

But the administrator realized something else. A true diplomat, he was heard to say only this of the incident: "Dr. Godley, ahem, strongly encouraged everyone to focus their attention on improving the way we conduct our affairs."

Well, it's true, isn't it? Dr. Godley certainly had focused everyone's attention. That was one of the things — one of the positive things — the administrator realized about this situation. He also understood that Dr. Godley had (perhaps unknowingly) handed him a ready-made, useful and wonderfully succinct goal statement.

What goal statement?

What others called "marching orders" were in fact a very clear statement of something that needed to be done at the clinic: get the doctor, the patient and the medical record in the same room at the same time.

You really have to admire how much that says in so few words, don't you?

The administrator had the statement printed and plastered up all over the staff areas of the clinic. Then he met with his key staffers and asked each of them to look at their work from the point of view of how to accomplish what Dr. Godley wanted. They outlined new procedures, defined employees' training needs, then trained them, and monitored their performance. And with their goal so clearly understood, guess what? They made remarkable progress towards achieving it! Morale improved, communication improved and lots of good things followed.

When our tactful administrator downplayed Dr. Godley's bad behavior, was he being generous? Sure. When he made certain the doctor's name appeared under the quotation on all the printed signs, was he being generous? Sure. But why not? He could afford to be generous. Dr. Godley had given him both the diagnosis and the prescription. All the administrator had to do was to make sure everybody took the medicine.

In the real world, viewing situations as problems will eat up your time and energy, often with no real solution. The problem you are trying to solve is often the symptom of a bigger problem. You have to make a conscious decision to view these situations as opportunities; when somebody brings you a "problem," think "opportunity"; look for the silver lining. When you train yourself to hear "opportunity" rather than "problem," all kinds of options are opened up to you beyond the immediate situation.

Competent administrators position themselves to step forward and take ownership and responsibility of "problems." Doing that practically guarantees opportunities for advancement. (Of course this presumes you figure out how to improve the situation. Here's a good rule: Pick your targets. It's up to you to assess the risks and gains of each situation that comes your way.)

When we advise people to equate problems with opportunities, we mean that literally. If you learn to hear "opportunity" every time someone says "problem," you will be amazed at the difference it makes.

People resist change. This includes most of your supervisors and superiors. But just let some huge, scary, hairy gorilla-of-a-problem show up at the doorstep. If you take charge of it and propose a solution, suddenly everyone starts scrambling to get on the "change" bandwagon. And who's going to be up there in the driver's seat of that bandwagon, smiling confidently and holding those reins like a natural-born 20-mule-team driver? You are. Congratulations!

Problems stimulate people to take action that they wouldn't take if there were no problem. That is where the opportunity comes from. This is a critical point to grasp: *when there are no problems, there are no opportunities*. Problems beget opportunities. In the absence of a problem, the status quo will almost certainly prevail.

Perception determines solution

Let's have another war story, and again look at it from both angles — problem and opportunity.

The situation: "Here they come again," thought Ms. Sharpe as Jane and Jim, the "front office fury and the front office fiend," charged toward her. It was not a new experience. Both of them wanted to run the department, and they would regularly move their tug of war into her office — after all, she was the administrator. Once there, they tugged, twisted, shouted, cussed, accused, denied, back-stabbed and contradicted as only two people committed to inflicting misery can do. Not getting anywhere with each other, they insisted she get involved.

Who gets the worst treatment in a tug of war? The rope does. It's in the mud from the start, and that's about the *best* it can hope for, because once the action begins the opposing forces will stretch and unravel and sometimes even break a rope. Ms. Sharpe was starting to feel like a rope.

This situation, viewed as a problem

Most of us don't even want to think about this "problem," much less become involved in it. It has pain written all over it. If we even acknowledge it, we then have to deal with issues such as the unacceptable behavior of the two employees; the effects of their running battle on medical staff and departmental staff and patients; the non-productive time spent fighting; the managerial need to assert authority and get Jane and Jim settled down, and on and on.

At the least, solving the "problem" will require the administrator to take an active role in the dispute, and might include disciplinary action against one or both employees, or even the suspension or termination of someone's employment.

Trying to find "solutions" to "problems" creates additional problems, such as possible EEO charges, lawsuits over termination, employees choosing up sides, low morale and perceptions of inept management for allowing the situation to develop in the first place.

This situation, viewed as an opportunity

Even though their competition was far from good-natured, it did help Ms. Sharpe realize that both Jane and Jim were capable of doing far more than was being asked of them. Yes, their behavior was unacceptable. But each needed to be in charge, and there was not enough work for the two of them to be in charge *of*. Ms. Sharpe heard opportunity knocking — the opportunity to get a lot more work out of two skilled and ambitious employees.

Jane in particular loved fast-paced, hectic work with lots of things to deal with at once. She had stated many times that she simply wanted to know what was expected of her and to be allowed to do it the way she thought was best for patients. She did not want anyone looking over her shoulder. She said she was responsible and she would do what it took to get the job done.

Ms. Sharpe asked Jane if she would like to turn her energy and determination to taking charge of something extremely important to the clinic, namely patient registration. Registration had been a problem for months and it was getting worse. And because registration controlled the work flow of others, it could have a major impact on efficiencies. Jane leaped at the opportunity. Her energy and imagination made an immediate difference in patient satisfaction and work flow. She became one of the happiest and most productive employees.

Jim was equally happy because the battle was over, leaving more time and energy to devote to the tasks he had charge of. Neither person was really furious or fiendish — they were frustrated. The key to eliminating the frustration was that, instead of believing their nasty bickering was a problem, Ms. Sharpe believed it was an opportunity. Instead of responding to the problem, which could only lead to more frustration, she chose to see it as an opportunity.

Like Ms. Sharpe, *your belief about similar situations absolutely determines the possible outcomes for them.* Seeing problems limits your solution to the terms of the problems. These solutions are usually win/lose outcomes. Someone must lose if you address the problem. Seeing opportunities opens possibilities for everyone to win.

Also, the person who sees opportunities is made more welcome than the one bearing problems. If you believe there are opportunities instead of problems, others will be eager to talk with you when you show up. Opportunities are more fun than problems. Here are some other common business situations that can be viewed as problems or as opportunities: computer crash, employee lawsuit, difficult patient, new government regulations, audits, books out of balance, strong new competition, just to name a few.

How do you approach things like these? How you view reality is to some extent a matter of choice. You take your choice and you pay your money. We know you have heard it another way, but this statement is more accurate. You choose to believe in problems or opportunities. Then you pay for your choice by the way you invest time, money and energy. If you invest in problems, the yield is limited. If you invest in opportunities, the yield can be much larger. Problems are often seen as insurmountable. But nobody thinks of an opportunity as "insurmountable" — your mind can't make those words fit together.

Opportunities are where you find them

Seeing opportunities where others see only problems will open up options beyond the immediate situation. In the previous case, had the administrator concentrated only on that rat's nest of problems, she might have missed a good opportunity for meaningful change. Don't avoid problems. On the contrary, smart administrators position themselves to step forward and take charge, to take ownership and responsibility, when problems arise — because that's when opportunity knocks.

Notice that a "rational" discussion and resolution of "the problem" did not occur in either war story. Good things happened in each case simply because individuals were committed to seeing opportunities, not problems. Perhaps this idea of personal commitment was stated best by Viktor Frankl, a psychotherapist. He spoke of being committed to finding the possibilities in even the most difficult situations and bringing those possibilities to life. He survived three Nazi concentration camps by viewing things from that angle.

We knew an Englishman who used to say, "Where there's muck, there's money." That thought is similar to our axiom about problems and opportunities. So is the fertilizer salesman's credo: "It may be manure to you, but it's my bread and butter."

Every black cloud disguises opportunities. The point of this chapter is that you are likely to find what you look for — look for problems and you will find them, look for opportunities and they will be there. You have to make a conscious choice to find those opportunities and focus on them. You have to make it a habit. Once you do, you will be amazed at the benefits you derive from simply changing your perspective.

Is Axiom 3, "You never have a problem — only an opportunity" a trite saying? Or is it a profound insight? Your habitual angle of view is a matter of personal choice and commitment. Your belief about Axiom 3 has enormous consequences for your career, and for other areas of your life as well.

To close this chapter and to make our final point about opportunities, let us quote a well-known and widely respected manager who lived a long time ago. You may have read about him in other books. His name was the Pied Piper, and here's what he was heard to say at a critical juncture in his career:

"Boy, that's a lot of rats! We really have a problem with these rats! (pause) But I wonder ..."

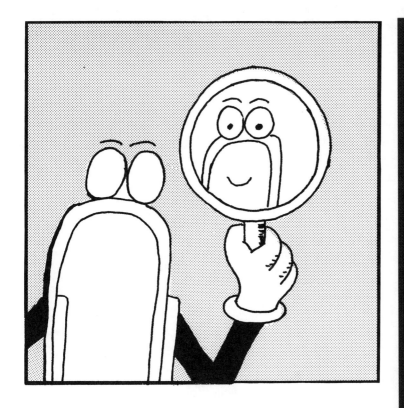

Look in the mirror, take a deep breath and count to ten

AXIOM 4

A bout half of the "funniest home videos" you see are pictures of kids, doing kids' stuff. Why are kids so much fun to watch? Lots of reasons, surely, but we're interested in a very unusual phenomenon: when you watch kids, your eyes see one thing but your brain sees another. Your eyes see what's happening at the moment, but your brain sees times past and times yet to come. It's as though you have a mirror on the past and a window to the future.

Watching kids, you can't help but reflect on how *you* looked and behaved at their age, and at the same time you can't help mentally rocketing these kids into the future, imagining how they will look and behave as they grow older.

It is easy to become introspective in moments like that, when you experience such an unusual breadth and clarity of vision. And it is exciting, because in those rare moments we often feel we are on the verge of understanding something important, of *comprehending*, of witnessing truth revealed.

Our discussions of timing, packaging, and problems vs. opportunities hinted at the fact that you — your motivations, your style, your emotions and other elements of *you* in the work place — are vitally important to your effectiveness and success. This chapter spells out the importance of *you.* You can understand the previous axioms perfectly and still fail completely because you don't understand *you* in the work place. This chapter is about perspective, about trying to see yourself as others see you, and trying to see

41

yourself accurately within the framework of your job and your career. We are going to focus on you.

Here it is, buck-naked, unadorned, blemishes and all: "*If you want to achieve success, go look in the mirror, take a deep breath and count to ten. You will see in the mirror everything you need to manage in order to achieve success.*"

Got a mirror handy? No? Use that mental mirror you're carrying. What? Oh, yes, everyone has a mental mirror. And a mental telescope, a periscope, a microscope, camera, tape recorder, spotlight, searchlight, flashlight, fog light, lie detector, stress analyzer, infrared night-vision goggles and so on. We've all got quite an array of instruments we can use for illuminating and analyzing subjects of interest, for detection and reflection, for "scoping things out," for measuring and evaluating the world around us.

In a moment we're going to suggest turning some of this equipment inward, using it to examine yourself. Many people cringe at that thought. "OH NO YOU DON'T!" is a common reaction. There, there. It'll be okay. Trust us — we work for doctors.

But first we have to tell you an unfortunate statistic: If you are like most people, a lot of your mental equipment is out of calibration. It hasn't been checked against reality for a long time. Worse, very little of it has ever been turned around to look inward, so the mechanisms probably need to be loosened and oiled before they'll swing around in that direction. And worst of all, if you're like most people, you have a little sign pinned up in your brain that says, "Safety first: Always wear rose-colored glasses when using this equipment for self-examination!"

Some of us have *prescription* rose-colored glasses ... and they're bifocals!

So we're going to ask you to take off the rose-colored glasses, get rid of the "fantasy filters" or anything else that might distort the truth, free up some of those powerful mental instruments, and take a good look at yourself.

Now you're asking if it will hurt. Well, yes, it might hurt a little, but it's good for you, so stop whining. Not to mention that doing this frequently and voluntarily is a lot better than being held up to a mirror by the scruff of the neck by external circumstances or, worse, by your superiors.

We will try to give you a reliable, non-distorting mirror in this chapter, to help you visualize some important things about yourself, and the effects those things may have on you, your people, and the organization.

The mirror won't help you if you don't take a deep breath, count to ten and really look. The mirror won't help you if you won't take a deep breath, count to ten and really look. The mirror won't help you if you won't take a deep breath, count to ten and really look.

Ready? Step up to the looking glass. The mirror we give you consists of a series of questions. It does not lead you into a wonderland. Quite the opposite. It removes the wonderland quality that distorts human interactions. It focuses on the pragmatic issues that you can change.

Do you understand the fundamental proposition?

In the introduction we mentioned "Critical Success Factors," the relatively few items essential to the survival of an enterprise. Now we're going to expand that thought a little, because we don't want our businesses merely to survive — we want them to thrive.

In medicine, "patient care" is always the goal. That's the way it should be. But in the day-to-day management of an organization, nobody deals with "patient care." What we deal with are the day-to-day issues and activities and people that *result* in patient care. We deal with scheduling, computers and telephones, reports, vendors, mail, government regulations and so on. So at any given moment, a good thing to ask is, "What's going on here? What are we working on right now, and why are we working on it right now?" In other words, what's the fundamental proposition?

Dr. Godley helped state a fundamental proposition succinctly when he said, "The object is to get the doctor, the patient and the medical record in the same room at the same time." That's something you can sink your teeth into, something you can roll up your sleeves and get to work on. If you had asked Dr. Godley, "What's the fundamental proposition today?" he'd tell you. He knew the answer.

And *you* should, too. Managers must first understand the core propositions of the business, and then organize people and processes to carry them out, tinkering constantly to keep things moving, and to keep molehills from turning into mountains. When you encounter mountains you must reduce them to molehills.

Look in the mirror. Do you have a good grasp of the fundamental business propositions for your organization? Have you organized in the best manner to carry them out? Do you know most of the ways things can go wrong, and do you have built-in methods to avoid them? Do you "tinker" and adjust as needed to keep things going along?

Most operations are like the lawnmower one of the authors used. It was never really broken and it was never really fixed. It required a lot of love and patience and constant tinkering with fuel mixture. However, out-of-pocket expenses for operation were only the cost of gasoline, a yearly oil change, and an occasional new spark plug. The lawnmower cut grass for 15 years, and the engine continues life as the power unit for a jury-rigged water pump, where it still sputters along. Not bad for a dysfunctional lawnmower.

Did a funny thing happen on the way?

Your present mood is a consequence of things that occurred earlier. During your reflective self-examinations, ask yourself what has happened up to this point in your day, week or month. Here are a couple of stories about managers having bad days, and about how they reacted to them.

Ms. Sharpe had inherited a situation not of her making and people not of her choosing. Key management persons and employees did not trust each other. She had spent many days trying to figure out how to reorganize the operation. She went to bed near midnight after a frustrating day and an inconclusive evening meeting. At 5 a.m. the next day she was awakened suddenly by a rude neighbor blowing his car horn. She knew she would not get back to sleep, so she decided to get up, read the paper and go to the office early. The paper had not arrived. She spilled coffee grounds, showered, cut herself while shaving and got her new hairdo wet. The paper still had not arrived. The cream was sour and the rolls were stale. She dropped her favorite coffee mug. Her belt broke, so she had to change suits.

By the time she arrived at the office, she had decided to clean house. She had decided to fire all the incompetent managers. She'd tell the others to cooperate or get out. She'd call a meeting and tell every last one of them in no uncertain terms that they must perform or face losing their jobs. She was fed up and was not going to take it any more.

You already know she didn't do those things. She took a deep breath and counted to ten. There were no firings or ultimatums. She realized that her day had just gotten off to a terrible start. She dug down and found some strength and patience. (For a manager, patience has to be like toothpaste in a tube: If you squeeze hard enough, you'll find there's always a little bit left.)

Unfortunately at that point she did what most of us do. She did not look in the mirror long enough. Her frustration burned in her stomach and had a bad effect on every conversation she had that day. Her people wondered why she was angry with them. When people wonder why, they fill in the blanks as best they can. Ms. Sharpe got herself functioning and avoided outright bloodshed, but she needed to spend more time analyzing what was happening to her and how she could best respond to it. She needed to spend more time looking in the mirror.

Another manager left the office for a lunch appointment. He had a flat tire on the way. It was 95 degrees, but in the interest of time, he changed the tire himself. He arrived late, hot and rumpled, with dirty hands and a streak of grime across his face. After lunch, he went to his car and found the spare tire he'd put on was now flat. No choice this time, call a service truck. As he waited for the truck in the shade of a tree, a bee flew up his pants leg. Stung him three times. The service truck driver inflated the tire and told the manager to follow him S-L-O-W-L-Y back to the tire store. The tire blew loudly just as they pulled in.

He arrived back at the office two hours behind in a full schedule of meetings. He was in an exquisitely foul mood. He walked in, called all the employees into his office, and said, "I am in a really bad mood. It is nobody's fault. Some things happened that shouldn't happen to a dog. I am frustrated and angry. Let's cancel our meetings this afternoon. If any of you need me for anything, I'll try to respond. If I snap at you, tell me I snapped, and I'll apologize. I'm going to close my door and enjoy my bad mood."

Within 45 minutes, he was feeling better. He went to a staff member and said, "We can talk about the project if you would like to, and please let me know if I'm not over my bad mood." They had a productive meeting and, buoyed by the improvement in his day, the manager chanced another and then another meeting, all of which turned out fine.

MORAL: It is okay to be human; it is not okay to inflict the pain of our humanity on others. Look in the mirror. Take a deep breath. Count to ten. See the human being there, as the second manager did. Accept your humanity, and let it work for you.

Because this manager was open and honest about his mood, his employees did not have to guess at the source of the problem, or wonder if they caused it. They did not walk around in fear that he would come down on them. Those are pretty good outcomes for a bad mood.

What is your emotional temperature?

When doctors do a physical examination they take "vital signs," including temperature. In this chapter we're proposing you do an examination of a different kind, but the concept of vital signs still applies. One of these vital signs is your emotional temperature. We'll talk about two indicators of temperature: first, emotions in general; and second, strong feelings about a particular issue.

Who are your favorite comic strip characters? The fat, wise-cracking, mischievous cat? The sleepy Army private? The soft-hearted Viking warrior?

What makes them interesting, and funny, and sometimes touching? One reason comic strips are so popular is that they reflect emotions in simple and obvious terms. But real people are usually harder to "read" emotionally than comic strip characters. And getting a good understanding of your own emotions can be surprisingly hard to do. Still, your success may depend on doing just that, because your emotions effect your behavior — and your behavior is what leads to success or failure.

Emotional energy is the source of creativity and accomplishment, as well as the source of destruction and frustration. We have no choice about emotions in the work place. Emotions are there, for all the good and all the ill that follow in their wake. But we do have a choice about what we *do* with our emotions.

Like comic strip characters, everyone has a habitual emotional state, a kind of balance point that they return to if their emotions have swung one way or the other. Some people are habitually lighthearted, some serious; some people are habitually sweet, some sour. In addition, some people display their emotions freely, while others cover them.

The point is that everyone — including you as a manager — acts on their emotions. This can be both a blessing and a curse.

Emotions are why we need the mirror. What we feel is a sane, rational, justified decision may appear insane, irrational and unjustified to others. In this chapter we are not too concerned about the decision itself; the issues here are the feelings, motives and emotions of you and the other people involved. Understanding these things is central to success in your career. In order to understand them you must learn introspection. In other words, you need to look inward, take a deep breath and count to ten.

A peer makes an excellent proposal. How do you react? Glad for the insights? Eager to cooperate? Jealous? Concerned about losing influence? What is your habitual emotional response? Look carefully in the mirror. We do not want to characterize the responses as positive or negative — every one of us is capable of responses ranging from admiration to jealousy. But we must evaluate the responses accurately. Greater awareness of our emotions leads to sharper insight about how they affect our behavior. Greater awareness of our emotions may even give us opportunities to adjust our behavior.

People tend to act out their feelings towards one another — although seldom as vividly as in the comics, thank goodness. Becoming aware of feelings gives you the opportunity to "edit" your behavior before things get out of hand or before you say or do something you might regret later.

Reflect for a minute on how you feel about the people you work with. Do you like them? Trust them? Feel they are competent? If your answer is consistently "no," might that say more about you than it does about them?

That is not a trick question and the answer is not always "yes." Some organizations populate themselves with incompetent, unlikable, untrustworthy people. Even if that is true, your feelings cannot become the issue. Regardless of how you feel, you must find ways to work effectively with others as long as all of you are in the organization.

A department supervisor insisted that the clinic administrator did not like him, even though the administrator consistently treated him with respect and evaluated him on the basis of performance against objectives. But the civility of their daily interaction did not alter the department supervisor's feelings. His own emotional temperature was cold and suspicious, and he perceived everything through the filter of those feelings. He made all facts fit the feelings, even if it required distorting the facts. And at some point, it was inevitable that he would begin to act on those feelings.

When you find yourself dealing with someone harboring such feelings, look in the mirror, take a deep breath and count to ten. At least one of you has feelings that are not grounded in reality, but that is not the point. What actually matters is that you understand the other person's feelings, and understand your own feelings, so you can use that insight to deal with the issue and improve the situation. You can change your behavior, if appropriate, with the idea of achieving a solid and practical working relationship.

Or you can make a big fuss, further alienating or even firing someone who may otherwise be a pretty good employee. Or you can let things smolder until they explode, and then wait to see if you'll find yourself answering charges of discrimination, harassment, unfairness. What a shame, because it is all needless. Remember, you'll see in the mirror everything you need to manage to enable everyone to win.

Still on the topic of emotional temperature, do you realize that your people accurately reflect your emotions? We do not mean they copy the emotions; they don't. What we mean is this: If your emotions inflict pain, your employees are likely to avoid you. If you are suspicious and hostile, your employees are more likely to treat patients and other employees the same way. If you explode over small things, your employees are more likely to do likewise. On the other hand, if you consistently show enthusiasm and openness, your employees will line up behind you and take their cues from you.

After all, you're the leader of your band, aren't you? Take charge! Put some zip in it! Managers manage. Leaders lead. If you're going to be a manager you've actually got to manage something. If you're going to be a leader you've got to *do some leading.* If you're going to get your people fired up, you've got to get fired up yourself.

What are your convictions?

Now, let's discuss strong feelings — another aspect of emotional temperature, but a little different from what we've been discussing, which was your overall, general or background emotional temperature. Keep in mind, the point of this chapter is to ask some questions about yourself. The answers to these questions can act as a "mirror" that may help you see yourself accurately within the framework of your job and your career.

We know a manager who simply stopped talking to a guy who worked for him when the employee let his hair grow long. The manager was offended by the employee's grooming, but that wasn't all; he believed long-haired men were unreliable. He felt very strongly about it. Without relating all the details, we will just say that as a result of the manager's shutting off communication with the employee, the company lost a large and important account.

Nothing shows the real you more clearly than the issues you feel strongly about. But more to the point, whenever you feel strongly about something, whenever you carry the torch for a particular cause, you can easily lose objectivity. Strong feelings are always warning signs.

We don't say you should be afraid to take a stand. On the contrary, you often have to take an enthusiastic stand on important issues. (In Dante's *Inferno* there was a special section, outside the gates of Hell, reserved for those who maintained their neutrality in times of crisis. These people were considered so loathsome that even the damned wouldn't mingle with them.) Our advice is not to be wishy-washy; our advice is to be careful. We want you to treat strong feelings as warnings to be careful.

One of the authors has a car with green, amber and red dashboard indicator lights. The green lights come on when things like cruise control or the high beams are in use. Green means "just a reminder." Amber lights come on for things like low fuel level or low washer fluid level. Amber means, "Hey, give this some thought." Red lights come on for serious conditions, like low oil pressure. Red means, "Pull over, now!"

When you have strong feelings on an issue, an amber light should glow on your mental dashboard, saying, "Hey, give this some thought." Why? Because strong personal feelings may cause you to see the issue incorrectly. You might lose perspective. You might relax your discipline. All of us are capable of snatching defeat from the jaws of victory.

The more strongly we feel about an issue, the less likely we might be to do the things essential to its success. Because the issue is so clear to us, we might be less likely to give others reasons for cooperating in terms of their own self interest: we'll assume they see the benefits as clearly as we do. We might be less likely to hear their concerns and questions as legitimate. We might be less likely to think critically about the issue. Often, the more heat there is on an issue, the less light there will be. More than at any other time, we need to take a deep breath and count to ten when we feel strongly about an issue. We really need to have a clear picture of ourselves and an accurate perspective of our surroundings at those times. Strong feelings can lead to inappropriate actions, and can produce exactly the opposite result we intend.

Here are some questions to ask yourself when you feel strongly about specific issues: Have I verified all the facts? Have I asked someone without an emotional stake in the issue to verify the facts and my reasoning? Have I given other people reasons *in terms of their self interest* to support my idea? Can I discuss the issue without my feelings dominating the discussion? Look into your mirror. If you are not sure, you may want to ask someone outside the situation to hold up their mirrors. Competent, trusted friends, consultants and professional counselors can be such resources.

So far we've asked three questions in our effort to create a mirror that helps you visualize yourself in your work. Here's the final question, one that puts some of your co-workers under the microscope.

Do you step into the spider's house?

"'Step into my house,' said the spider to the fly." We all know the spider wishes to catch the fly in its web and eat it alive. That story is an apt analogy of what happens to us when we get caught up in the webs others may spin. In your reflective moments, when you are trying to see yourself accurately within your work environment, check to be sure you are not caught in webs of emotion or office politics.

Do you have spiders at work in your organization? Absolutely. And sharks, vultures, Venus fly-traps and lions and tigers and bears — oh, my! It might be fun to make point-for-point comparisons between people in our organizations and predators found in nature, but for now it's enough to say this: Look in the mirror — is what you see there someone else's lunch?

In daily interactions between people, where does "influence" end and "manipulation" begin? Tough question. We don't have the answer. We know, though, that managers must exert influence in order to be effective in their jobs. And we know that most people are also capable of manipulation. Manipulative people are like spiders, spinning webs to trap their victims.

Interestingly, just as in nature, some office spiders act purely on instinct, habitually spinning webs, mindlessly feeding on their prey. Simple example: All of us know employees who never tire of saying things like, "Everyone makes fun of me. They all go on coffee break together and plan how to make me do all the work while they goof off." The statement might have a basis in fact, or it might not. It doesn't matter: non-specific accusations are a trap. Call this "The web of suspicion."

What the employee wants you to do is the same thing children want you to do when they tattle on each other: they want you to grab the offenders and punch their livers out. Minimum. Or at the very, *very* least, you are expected to stomp around and scare the living daylights out of 'em.

As a manager you must, of course, deal with the employee's feelings — which may be the most important issue anyway. But you mustn't pre-suppose anything, and you mustn't minimize the importance of the actual complaint. Just don't fall into the trap. Take a deep breath and count to ten. Tell the employee that you will not allow anyone to treat another unfairly. Tell them you are poised for action. And then tell them this: in order to act, you must have clear instances of specific behaviors.

Ah, but the spider does not want to deal with facts; the spider wants us caught in the web. Take a deep breath, count to ten and talk with them about the necessity of performing the job. If the employee says, "I can't do my job when people work against me," take a deep breath, count to ten and say this: "We will not allow unfair treatment. We must have clear examples of specific behavior in order to take action." *

You can play that response like a broken record. You can say that continuing to complain about others without clear instances of specific behaviors is not acceptable. Do not be surprised if this employee becomes very angry when you do not get caught up in the emotions. In fact, expect it, and prepare for a formal complaint by documenting your conversations and having a superior review them. People who spin webs can take them dead seriously.

Remember the department supervisor who insisted the clinic administrator did not like him? The fact that he was a minority employee over age 40 complicated the issue. The only way to deal with the issue was in terms of performance against the job requirements. The clinic administrator actually had a high opinion of the supervisor's abilities. Did the clinic administrator "like" him? It's irrelevant. Liking someone is not a job requirement. Working together effectively is. Yet "liking" was the issue the supervisor returned to again and again. Why?

Figure it out. "Liking" is an emotionally-charged, irrelevant issue. It can't be quantified easily. It is a problem without a resolution. It's sticky. Sticky like tar. Sticky like a spider's web. The real issue, as you will see in a later chapter, is power. The trap was "The web of power."

You can fall into lots of different traps. We've seen two so far, and you could probably think of two dozen. They'll resemble each other, with things like "suspicion" and "power" forming the strands of the web, and emotions like "anger" and "anxiety" acting as the sticky goo the strands are covered with. Anger and anxiety are contagious. When an employee charges into your office in anger, whatever the issue is, take a deep breath and count to ten. If you get caught up in the emotion, you have no chance of discovering the facts. You'll waste time and energy and perhaps act inappropriately. Deal with the emotions as presented, but without getting caught up in them.

---

*Note that there are times when legally you must act based on feelings or allegations reported to you. For example, when you are told of possible illegal discrimination or sexual harassment.

Getting caught up in these webs causes you to lose not just time and energy, but also credibility as a leader. You lose the opportunity to help others gain a perspective beneficial to themselves as well as to the organization. Luckily, there are warning signs next to most traps. The warning signs are displays of strong feelings — your own, or someone else's.

In highly emotional confrontations, one manager we know stays calm, listens carefully, and says, "I ain't gonna put my dog in that fight, and here's why." He then outlines what is acceptable and what is not acceptable job-related behavior, and he asks for cooperation. It almost always works. Employees who do not cooperate will have a conversation with him on the topic of "How much do I value my job?"

Isn't that better than stepping into the spider's house?

Making self-assessment easier

One of the authors likes to cook. His beginning point is that you cannot make the quality of a meal any better than the quality of the raw product — you can only maintain it or make it worse.

To many of your employees, you are the raw material of your projects. In other words, your projects are only as good as you are, as a boss and as a human being. Now, is this realistic? Is it true? No. Bad people can have good ideas; good people can make bone-headed mistakes. You can't judge a book by its cover. Yet the perception is very widespread that if you yourself are tarnished in some way, your ideas and proposals are likewise tainted.

Take a deep breath and count to ten. Look hard at what you do and why you do it. And look very hard at what people perceive you to do and why they perceive you to do it. The only way to affect their perceptions is to change what you see in the mirror.

Yes, yes, we know; we keep telling you to manage others by managing yourself. Like charity, management begins "at home."

We started this chapter by saying it might hurt a bit to take a long, hard look at yourself, and that despite your other abilities you can fail completely because you don't understand and manage **you** in the work place. In the final analysis, the greatest management challenge is that of managing yourself. Here are two techniques for making self-assessment less difficult.

Reflect on yourself regularly

The first technique is to make and keep a regular appointment with yourself. Spend at least an hour a week reflecting on what you are doing and why you are doing it. Ask questions that lead to other questions, such as: What are my motivations? What do others perceive my motives to be? Do I focus on what I can change in me, instead of concentrating on what others do that I find frustrating? Am I just doing the same thing every day the same way? Do I need to be less changeable? Do I need to be more changeable? Am I willing to consider that I could be completely wrong on an issue? How do I react to anger?

Borrow another person's mirror. Look at your behavior through the eyes of other persons, especially those you don't see eye-to-eye with. A test of your maturity as a manager is your ability to get outside your own frame of reference. It is also good discipline. Ask yourself, "If I were John, how would I react to my proposal?" Doing that can give insight into how to work more effectively with John, and it shows us the holes in our own work. People who react negatively to us do us a great service. They give us clear feedback.

Treat frustration and anger as friends, not enemies. Think of them as a red light glowing on the dashboard — a signal to pull over to stop and think about what you do and why you do it. Anger and frustration signal us that another motivation is about to impose itself on us. That knowledge empowers us to act more constructively.

Network with people you trust

The second technique to make your self-examinations less painful is not to do them by yourself. Develop a network of people you trust, people who will act in your best interests. That may include reflecting back to you some things about yourself that you don't want to see. Be thankful for the feedback. Trusted, competent friends outside your organization can be advocates for you, and you can return the favor for them.

Management requires a delicate balancing act. We must be willing to stake our careers on a direction, and be willing to abandon it on short notice when it becomes clear that things have changed.

We must be sure enough to act without second-guessing ourselves, and we must be willing to entertain ideas that contradict what we intend to do. Given the stresses of that challenge, it is no wonder that we find comfort in acting impulsively or in doing the same thing the same way every day. Both are traps. Looking in the mirror, taking a deep breath and counting to ten, is the way to avoid those traps, and to manage around our own imperfections and the imperfections of others.

Because we are human, there are some days when we should not attempt anything that can be fouled up. When employees have those days, one of the kindest things we can do is transfer them to something they can't foul up, send them on an errand, or just say, "You seem to be struggling, why not walk away from it for a while and take an extra break?" And sometimes the kindest thing you can do for yourself is to isolate yourself in your office for awhile. Just walk in and close the door behind you. The world will still be there when you come out.

Final thought

In addition to burdening you with some heavy philosophy, in this chapter we went poking around in your brain, and we found things like mirrors, microscopes, tape recorders, rose-colored glasses, fantasy filters and dashboard lights. You really ought to do something about all that stuff cluttering up your mind. We think you need a vacation!

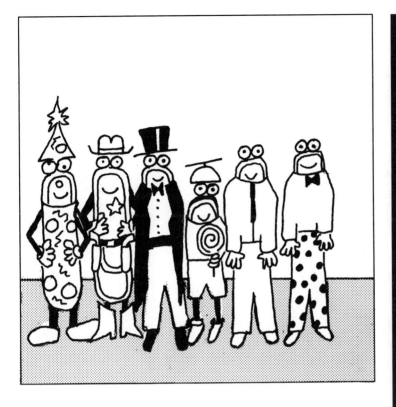

There are different strokes for different folks

AXIOM 5

T he classic advertising photograph of an amusement park roller coaster shows two riders in the front compartment. The coaster is cresting a hill, at the point where gravity seems to lose its grip. The guy on the left is having a completely wonderful time. Courting danger, he has his hands up in the air. He's enjoying the thrills of speed and weightlessness. He has an enormous smile on his face.

The person on the right is not smiling. You can see the frown on his lips, but you can't see the terror in his eyes, because he's covering his eyes with one hand. The other hand grips the safety bar ferociously. He is completely terrified. He thinks he's going to die. He's pretty sure he's going to die in the next three seconds. If you were sitting three seconds from eternity, would you look happy? Of course not. He doesn't, either; he looks miserable.

How can this be? On the same day, at the same amusement park, on the same roller coaster — in the same *seat*, for goodness sake — one rider is having the best time of his life, yet the other rider is having the worst time of his life. How do you explain that?

There's only one answer: different strokes for different folks.

In this chapter, we talk about the enormous variety of needs and desires people bring with them to the work place. We'll talk about you and the people you work with. We will present a recipe for the brew of human interactions. We will define the major ingredients and discuss their effects. And we'll give you some practical tips for dealing with, and even enjoying, this potent brew.

Here's our premise: People act in usual patterns of behavior they have developed over time. These patterns seem right and feel right to them, and give them comfort. Also, people feel uncomfortable with challenges to these patterns. The circumstances that create comfort in one person can create discomfort in another. The very situation that makes one person productive immobilizes another — just like the roller coaster.

A quick story:

Jack's boss wanted him to take on more responsibility. Jack was a moderately competent supervisor, and the boss thought surely Jack wanted more freedom and responsibility and certainly wanted to avoid those unpleasant times when she had to "fuss" at him. Yet the more responsibility she gave him, the worse Jack performed. She coached him on planning, time management and guidelines for decisions. Jack could replay it all to her without error, but would always manage to foul up again and again.

Finally, the foul-up that could not be ignored. Jack caused an emergency on a Saturday, and the boss had to return to work from a week-end outing to repair the damage. Come Monday, she called Jack to her office and gave a thoroughly pointed and exquisitely descriptive narration of his shortcomings, her anger and the consequences of any similar foul-ups in the future. The sharper her comments became, the more Jack leaned forward and seemed to relax. Then it occurred to her — Jack found the increased freedom and responsibility she had given him paralyzing. And ironically, after being given more freedom, Jack now felt less important than before, because he was getting less attention.

After the upbraiding, Jack left the office his old moderately competent self, which was more than acceptable for his position. His department worked okay — not great, but okay. The boss made a mental note to call Jack in once a month, even if she had to make up something to complain about. That was the only way Jack felt appreciated. It worked like a charm from then on. And although this particular brew was unusual, it was satisfying and workable.

The main ingredients

Watching people interact in the work place can call to mind an image of a big pot brewing and bubbling on the stove. There are at least four major ingredients that go into the brew: feelings, process, results and power. Everyone attempts to combine these ingredients in a mixture that sits well with them. The problem is that the recipe that satisfies one person gives another indigestion and may poison a third. At the deepest level of our *selves*, there are truly different strokes for different folks. What gives one person a "good, warm feeling" alienates another. Jack experienced a chewing out as a form of care. Others experience it as a form of aggression. It is important — critically important — to recognize such variations in people's perceptions and preferences, to understand which "ingredients" they like, which they can tolerate, which they simply can't abide.

How do you tell? The easy way is to ask. Ask solid, open questions. Ask, "How do you feel about that?" "What's your opinion?" "Do you think this will work?" "What's wrong with this plan?" "Do you want to tackle this?" Then be quiet and pay attention to what they tell you. Usually people will make their own perspectives clear — if you're smart enough to listen.

Let's now look at these basic ingredients in human behavior and how to spot them in day-to-day actions.

Feelings

First, feelings. A person we knew quit smoking after 20 years of three packs a day. One day, he sat hunched over his desk, face screwed into deep concentration, eyes bulging out and fists clinched into white knuckles.

"What are you doing, Joe?"

"I'm not smoking a cigarette, that's what I'm doing."

Now Joe was a "feelings" guy, and if you knew that you would see he was acting in character. Joe would act when things felt right — and not a moment sooner. It is easy to become involved in monumental struggles with these people, because their resistance increases exponentially with the amount of logic, persuasion and power that others apply. None of that matters, because they won't budge until it feels right.

How do you recognize someone who acts on feelings? Watch and listen for two clues. First, their positions are often self-validating: things are true or right or proper because this person *feels* them to be so. Their refrain is "I don't feel right" about this or that. The second clue is that they often convert discussions into whether or not you like them. They need — they really *need* — to feel right about the whole ball of wax. It is difficult for them to comprehend the thought of people working well with others they don't particularly like.

Process

Second, process. A consultant we know interviewed a department store clerk who spent three hours a day copying information from papers onto 3" x 5" cards, which she then filed alphabetically. He didn't see any purpose for the task — it turns out that there was no worthwhile purpose — so he asked, "Why do you do that?"

"I copy the listed items that are missing from the papers and file them under the person's name."

"How long have you done that?"

"For two years," she said.

"What do you do as a result of filing these cards?"

"I don't do anything."

"What would happen if you quit doing this?"

"Mr. Brane told me to do it. I'm sure he has a reason; I would be afraid to stop."

Her major ingredient was process. She felt comfortable following process. She did not feel comfortable questioning it or changing it. Such persons have faith that by doing the process properly, one step at a time, everything will turn out all right. They get to the result by following the process.

The sure way to create havoc for persons whose primary focus is process is to ask them to change without giving them good reasons for the change and plenty of time to change. Ask them to create a new process, and they may resign. But, if you need someone to follow the processes exactly — for example, in the lab, medical records or billing — this clerk would be a good employee. She did what she was asked. The problem was not hers. The problem was with the lack of adequate management instruction. Such people are valuable. Get too many of them, however, and every change becomes a wrestling match.

Results

Jonathan and his father, the farmer, were building a new barn. It was an ecologically correct barn, with the roof being made from recycled corrugated tin roofing from an old barn they had demolished. The only problem was that the old tin sheets were not long enough. One sheet wouldn't reach from the peak to the bottom of the roof; one and one-half lengths of the old material were required. If you've never cut corrugated tin roofing with handshears, it is difficult to appreciate the challenge. The father got two burst blisters and three cuts on his wrist, and he used his entire vocabulary just to cut one sheet of tin. Only nine more to go.

"Say, dad?" Jonathan asked, "Since we need a 'half sheet' on every strip, why don't we take a full sheet and bend it over the peak. That way half of it will be on each side, and we won't have to cut it."

"It won't work, Jonathan," the dad said. "I buy your books and send you to school, and you don't learn any more than that?"

Jonathan thought, but did not say, "Dad doesn't have enough skin to cut another sheet, and he has already gone past 'dad-gum' to 'frazzlin tin shears,' so he is out of bad words. I'll just wait." (Jonathan had learned more than his dad realized.) In a few minutes, his dad said, "What was that silly idea of yours?" In slightly more time than it took to cut the first sheet, they finished the roof. It did not leak. A leak-free roof was the result they wanted.

Jonathan and his father were in the classic process-versus-result conflict. Jonathan was mostly interested in the result, and would invent the process required to get it. (Jonathan was mostly interested in finishing the roof so he could visit Julie on the next farm, which was the *real* result he was after.) Jonathan's dad appreciated results, but was a "process" man; placing his trust in the process, he knew that if he just went about his work in the proper way, the result was guaranteed. He took "process" a little more seriously than Jonathan, and wanted to roof that barn the right way. But under pressure he was willing to negotiate on the process in order to get the result of a waterproof roof at minimum expense.

The best part of that story is that both had become astute enough along the way not to offend the other's preferred style, and astute enough to recognize that each had an understanding the other lacked. They trusted each other to do what it took to keep the farm operating, and they could banter about their differences.

People whose major ingredient is results can make things happen. The down side is that they often make the wrong things happen or make unintended things happen. Why? Because they don't spend enough time with process to ensure getting the result they want. Jonathan once shocked himself with 110 volts by trying to rig up an electric worm digger without bothering to understand the processes for working safely with electricity. He did it only once. Next time he decided to study the process.

Power

The fourth ingredient is power. This topic is dealt with extensively in the next chapter, but we can make a few observations here.

Some people bring power as the major ingredient to the brew of human relationships. They do not depend on process, feelings or anything except power to get things done. Ask them to drive a tack, they will use a sledge hammer. Suggest competition, they will bury you. Their credo is, "I will make it work." And they do, most of the time, until they run into someone who has more power.

People who operate from a basis of power create a kind of gunslinger stand-off time after time. Everything comes down to a one-on-one contest. Some managers enjoy power so much that everything they say is issued as an order. Some employees have discovered the power of resistance, and use it to drive their managers to tranquilizers.

Now, don't get us wrong: the use of power is required for anything to get done. Power will be exercised in human activities — that's for sure, and it is not a bad thing. But the trick is to use power appropriately and intelligently. The trick is to gain power by giving power — in other words, to share power.

Read the labels

Obviously, nobody's approach to something will be 100 percent feelings, process, results, power or anything else. We are all a mixture of things. As a manager, the point is not to violate other people's sense of comfort. Not violating comfort, rather than trying to "act like" what you think the person wants, is the key to a successful relationship.

Now, some specific observations:

• Most people want their work situation to meet their needs, and they want to be in charge of their own destiny at work. They will strive for that, using an approach that emphasizes feelings, process, results or power;

• Some ingredients have built-in conflicts with others. For example, individuals who are oriented toward power often do not trust either process or feelings;

• Some ingredients have built-in trust. For example, results-oriented people and power-oriented people tend to trust (not necessarily like) each other, as do process-oriented and feelings-oriented people; and

• Conflicts more often grow out of the differences in the mix of ingredients than out of the stated issue. Situations can almost always be improved with dialogue that seeks to appreciate the style, the perspective, the comfort level and the preferences of others.

Speaking of conflicts, when you turn up the heat, the brew thickens in several ways. The primary ingredient may become more pronounced, or another ingredient can become dominant. Under pressure, some people change their position and their approach to getting things done. Also, surprise ingredients may pop up and change the brew.

Let's spend some time on the topic of conflict, because in the practical world "different strokes" means conflict is inevitable.

The 100 proof brew

One of the authors got a speeding ticket not long ago. It's a terrific story, and if this were a novel, the climactic moment would look something like this:

> The trooper's voice rose a notch in pitch and two notches in volume. He bit off the words and spit them at me:
>
> "So, you don't think I know what I'm doing, and you think I'm dishonest?"
>
> "No," I said. "I simply want to know the process of calibrating the radar."
>
> His face turned a deep red as he ripped the citation out of the book and threw it at me.
>
> "You'll find that out in court." His hand drifted down toward his gun. Now, I was scared. "Get moving," he hissed.

The writer felt he'd had a narrow escape. Something really went wrong. A routine conversation almost turned into a fearful incident.

Think of the times when things go wrong in your clinic or office or hospital. You are going along just doing your job. Out of the blue, without warning, an employee angrily confronts you with a surprise grievance. Normally-cooperative individuals surprise you with resistance. An employee you thought enjoyed working with you recites a litany of your failures and suggests you can't be trusted. One peer says you move too fast; another says you move too slow. Too many details, according to some. Too few details, according to others. You run over feelings, some say. You let feelings keep you from moving, others say.

These situations can feel a lot like the author's speeding ticket incident. Things go badly wrong. Feelings rise, heels dig in and participants look for ammunition to defend themselves and to fire at others. What should be routine exchanges can escalate into warfare of some type. Usually the conflicts are played out politically, or in some other socially acceptable way. Sometimes, though, they explode into real physical violence. Most work place violence with firearms began with routine exchanges. We must not ignore that possibility. In any case, people get hurt, careers go off track and organizations become dysfunctional or even go out of business, because of failures to communicate and failures to understand other people's needs.

What goes wrong? The same thing that goes wrong in every situation of conflict. The very factors that create comfort and efficiency in one person create discomfort and inefficiency in another. On the same day, in the same office, with the same elevator music playing in the background, mix radically different reactions to the same factors in any situation and conflict has to emerge. Throw some tension in the pot, add a little fatigue and stir in some resentment. The resulting brew cooks out to about 100 proof. But it is like the old moonshiner in Arkansas said. "I know it's a hunderd proof; I just ain't sure what it's a hunderd proof of."

What cooks out depends on the mix of ingredients and who stirs the pot. People in authority, like you, have big spoons. We stir the pot, and we affect how every other person stirs the pot. The trooper's approach affected the manner of the questions, which in turn affected the motorist's responses, which affected the following questions, which affected the following responses, and so on. And we mentioned surprise ingredients, didn't we? The brew of human relationships always contains surprise ingredients such as the motivations and the instability of those involved.

You may not always be able to cook up a brew you want, but you can frequently keep it from becoming a brew that you don't want. It is possible to manage conflict and prevent a lot of damage. It is possible to limit the damage when things go wrong between people.

A radar detector might have warned of the patrolman's presence in the story of the speeding ticket. But you don't need "radar" to detect the signals from others at work. You do have to be willing to read the signals they give and understand what they mean. Pay attention. There are usually plenty of advance indicators.

Still on the topic of conflict, how can you keep the brew from becoming explosive? Here are some simple guidelines:

- Give your word and keep it. It is important for others to know that your "yes" means yes and your "no" means no. Don't give your word if you are not sure you can keep it. "Trust me" cuts it only after you establish a track record of trustworthiness — and by then you don't have to say it;

- Create relationships of value. People who value relationships will protect them, overcome conflict and negotiate win/win outcomes. People who do not value their relationships fight over everything;

- Practice "playback listening." Consciously listen to the words of others, then play back what they said. The playback includes facts and feelings. "Dr. Able, I want to make sure I understand the outcomes you expect. You expect that we will use the new consent form by Monday and we should not worry about the expense of hurry-up printing. Did I get the sense of what you said?" You might also ask another to play back what you said. "Joan, I need to make sure I said what I meant to say. Play back to me what you are going to do about the new consent form." If the playback is not what you meant to communicate, say so. Say, "Well, I didn't say what I meant to say. Let me try again."; and

- Be alert for reactions that are out of proportion, and back off. An office manager asked an outside computer specialist to install software on her computer. When the specialist asked her to enter her password to begin the installation, she became livid. She said he should know how to do it himself, and that she would not have called him if she had known he was incompetent. She said the software probably would not work, and if it did work it would be more trouble than it was worth. She said he represented himself dishonestly, and that everyone she worked with thought the same;

Obviously she over-reacted. Something else was on her mind. Reactions that do not fit the situation tell us to quit stirring the pot. The patrolman signaled the surprise ingredient of instability when he threw the citation and let his hand drift to his revolver; clearly it was time to quit stirring the pot, regardless of any constitutional right to do so.

The point is to use caution when people behave inappropriately. As business people we cannot and should not make judgments about the stability of others — at least not for conversation. Those judgments might create more fights (including legal fights) than can be managed. If people do not give their word and keep it, and if they react out of proportion, be on the lookout for surprise ingredients. Caution is in order.

We've spent some time on the topic of conflict, but as managers we must strive not merely to reduce conflict, but also to increase co-operation. That is the topic of the next section.

Nicer thoughts and recommendations

It is clear that people bring a variety of desires, needs and expectations with them to work. Great. So how does that help you as a manager? What do you *do* with that knowledge?

Use it. Apply it. Derive some practical advantage from it.

How, specifically? Hire a consultant. Do some personality profiling, training and team-building. Then roll up your sleeves and get to work.

Oh, no! We said "personality." The "P" word.

Why are many managers afraid of personality profiling? Probably because of the "H" word — hogwash. An enormous amount of hogwash has been disseminated on this topic. Or the "M" word — manipulation. Trying to figure out someone's personality type seems tricky and manipulative to many people.

Let's cut through some of this.

Of all the things we rely on as managers, we rely on people more than anything else. Of all the things we use to get our work done, we use people more than anything else. Yes, we "use" people, in the very healthiest sense of that word. We can't avoid it, and shouldn't try. Instead, we should strive to use our employees fittingly, and properly, and well. To do that we should make a serious effort to see them as human beings, and to help them see us and each other in that same light. We should try to gain insight into how to work with people whose outlooks and needs are different from our own.

Saying that is easy. Doing it is a lot harder, primarily because of the hogwash factor involved. But that is no excuse for not trying. If you're not an expert on this topic, shop around among consultants or specialists and find someone you feel comfortable talking with. Spend some money on this. Get with a program. Again, to repeat the advice: Hire a consultant. Do some personality profiling, training and team-building. Then roll up your sleeves and get to work.

Summary

There are different strokes for different folks. What frees one person, immobilizes another. What makes one feel good makes another feel bad. What builds trust and cooperation in one destroys it in another. The volatile brew of human relationships can be productive and fun, if we go to the trouble of recognizing and responding appropriately to the people involved. The single greatest management failing is the failure to do so. If you've ever overindulged on a favorite food, you know the meaning of the expression "too much of a good thing." In the brew of human interactions, each ingredient brings something unique, and the brew benefits from the variety. All the ingredients are needed. If any one ingredient dominates, no matter how worthwhile it is, it will probably be "too much of a good thing."

As managers we stir the pot and mix the ingredients according to our personal tastes. That tendency is both right and human. But we must expand our tastes, and strive to appreciate the rich variety of flavors to be found in the larger world. This requires discipline and effort, but the rewards are immense.

Final thoughts

We opened this chapter by talking about a roller coaster at an amusement park. We don't mean to suggest your place of business is like an amusement park — really, we don't. And we're not trying to compare your job to a roller coaster ride — really, we're not. Using the literary technique of "metaphor" would be out of place in a book like this, don't you think? Besides, your office is not an apt metaphor for an amusement park: At the amusement park *you pay* to have fun, whereas at work, *they pay you* to have fun. Really, they do!

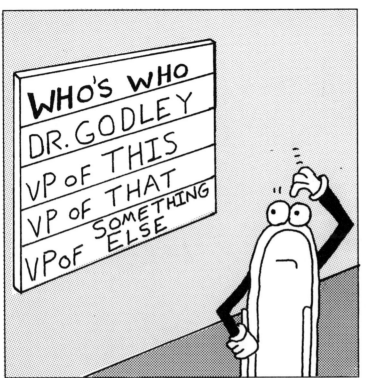

Know who is boss, and count your votes

"We'll just find out who's the human resources director of this hospital — her or
me!" Rich growled as he charged toward
the president's office.

"Wait a minute," you say, "I've never
seen you like this! What's going on?"

"One of the supervisors wants to promote Sally to the reception
area on the executive floor. Sally wants the promotion and I
approved it."

You reply, "That's standard procedure ... so why are you upset?"

"Marilyn heard about it, and called to tell me that she doesn't
want Sally working on her floor."

Marilyn is the long-term, somewhat cantankerous secretary to
one of the partners, a physician who had no policy, management or
operational responsibilities.

"Rich, wait! You need to know who's ..." Rich leaves your words
hanging in air and charges down the stairs two at a time.

You run into a much-less-lively Rich an hour later in the coffee
shop. He looks chastened and deflated — like somebody had
knocked the wind out of him. He says, "Well, I found out who's
Human Resources Director ... Marilyn is. Sally can't work on her
floor." Rich just learned about Axiom 6 the hard way.

"Know who's boss." Nobody really argues with that concept. The
real trick is to know *how* to know who's boss. That's what we cover
in this chapter, along with how to "count your votes."

Rich made the mistake of confusing the organization chart with the real power structure in an organization in a specific situation. Clearly, Marilyn was the boss in that situation. Knowing who's boss is knowing about power: who has it and when.

Why did Marilyn have that power? Her boss gave it to her. Why did her boss have power? Because he was a partner, a physician and a good friend of some of the hospital's top admitters. Any one of those reasons is sufficient. So when Marilyn told her boss she didn't think Sally would fit in on the first floor, her boss told the president, and the president told Rich, and Sally was not promoted.

Wait a minute, that's not fair. Right! That is abuse of power. Perhaps. Something should be done about it. Maybe — but maybe not.

Power. It's like the air we breathe. Creative and humane uses of power refresh us as much as the sweetness of a deep breath in the early morning. Whimsical, destructive uses of power can make us feel like we've been punched in the belly. Like we've had the wind knocked out of us.

Power is the ability to get things done, to stop things from being done, or to reverse a decision about what is to be done. The person who owns the power in a situation is the boss. As the hospital's human resources director in the story above, Rich certainly had power. But he wasn't the boss in the situation presented.

The story illustrates a common human experience — the arbitrary exercise of power. Rich was lucky. He learned who was boss in that situation. He learned it a little late, but he learned it in time to limit the damage. He got out of it with frustration, a bruised ego and an employee named Sally who wondered what the heck was going on. He could have damaged his career by insisting that the president deal with the unfairness. He stared power in the face and had to blink.

We are not going to look for any justification for the shabby treatment Sally got, nor will we claim Marilyn should have a conscience or that her boss should have a backbone. We won't even suggest that the president should have backed Rich. All those statements may be true, but they are not relevant.

We *are* going to assert that Rich could have and should have prevented the entire ugly encounter by knowing who was boss. Had Rich known who was boss, he could have avoided embarrassment,

Sally's hurt feelings, and the delay in filling an important administrative position. Had Rich known who was boss he would have been a better manager.

Here are some guidelines for how to know who's boss. These cover such things as understanding how power is used in your organization, sharing power with peers and employees, and knowing when to put up and when to shut up.

Understand the Golden Rule

The Golden Rule is: "The person with the gold makes the rules." Corny and contrived, but true.

"Gold" is whatever someone has that someone else wants. At any time on any issue, somebody probably has something that someone else wants, and that puts one of them in a more powerful position than the other.

It's not really all that hard to figure out who has the power, if you're observant and willing to do some simple analysis. For example, in the hospital story, Rich had never before been asked to approve a transfer to the reception area. He would have been well advised to scout the territory in advance. He should have done some sniffing and snooping, some exploring, some surveying; he should have gotten the lay of the land.

Instead, he got blindsided. He got hit from the flank when he charged in after encountering resistance. He rushed in, when he should have stepped gently.

When you are wondering who's boss, keep in mind the obvious fact that money very often conveys power with it. People who have spending authority have power. These are usually the people way up on the organization chart. But also look for the person who has "the power of the purse strings." Fairly often you find powerful individuals who do not have spending authority, but who can limit appropriations or can veto expenditures. These are sometimes comptrollers or budget officers, whose organizational positions might not be lofty, but who can quickly reel in your high-flying plans.

"Veto power" is a type of gold. If you want something, and someone else can prevent you from getting it even if they don't have it themselves, they've got power you have to deal with.

Kinship, personal friendships and debts of all kinds are gold. Did you just get a new job? Find out immediately who's related to whom, and who is friends with whom. There's gold in those hills.

It's really not that hard to figure out who has power. True, it is sometimes hard to imagine *why* somebody has power. ("Wonder why Marilyn makes a good salary by doing so little?") But even though that can be an interesting topic, it's probably not important. In the practical world you have to deal with things you can't change, and the structure of power in your organization is most likely one of those things.

Know how your organization uses power

There are two basic approaches to using power. In one, power is concentrated within the smallest number of people possible. Those in the nucleus make all the decisions. This approach to power may grow out of the need to keep operations simple, or to ensure coordination, or to control expenses. Let's face it, a business with an autocratic and controlling boss can operate with less skilled (and therefore less costly) employees in most positions, and may be more profitable than a competitor that has more of the higher-paid employees.

The contrasting approach is to share power broadly. Top management develops a cadre of self-motivated and competent managers who operate independently within the guidelines they helped create. In this approach, managers are encouraged to assess and take intelligent risks and be accountable for their decisions. Let's face it, personnel costs can be higher, coordination can be more difficult, and there are more ways to foul up under this approach to power.

Neither approach to power is right, and neither approach is wrong. Either can work well — although these days most people pray at the Shrine of Shared Power, and regard concentrated power as devil-worship. Sharing power seems somehow more humane and more fair than concentrating power. But, neither system is inherently good or bad, right or wrong, humane or inhumane. Each one works, if that is the way the organization shares power.

The point is that part of "knowing who is boss" is knowing how your organization shares power. Trying to buck the approach your organization uses is a sure-fire recipe for frustration. To assume power is available for sharing, in a place that uses the concentrated power approach, is asking for ulcers. In those places, the senior executives want to make all the decisions. Period. They've nailed the lid shut on the suggestion box, and they've scribbled the words "Don't bother" to the cheery little sign that says "Give us your suggestions!"

That's not a joke: everyone would be better off if there *were* such a sign. That way everyone would understand the deal, and would know what to expect. The power structure would be perfectly clear. People could take it or leave it. Nothing wrong with that, is there?

But lots of executives want to be *regarded* as power-sharing kinds of people, even when they're not. Most people, including CEOs, don't like to be called autocratic devil-worshippers. So they masquerade and equivocate, when straight-in-the-eye honesty would be a better policy — as it usually is.

Know when to put up

A bunch of us farm boys used to dare one another to do silly or dangerous things, and as collateral for the bet we'd "put up" something we treasured. "I'll put up my pocket knife and dare you to eat six raw eggs," meant if you ate the eggs, you got the knife.

"Putting up" always took place within the context of a contest or a challenge. Somebody had a point to prove. Somebody wanted to demonstrate superiority. Somebody wanted to be boss. As a manager you may sometimes have to put up. The managerial game is played with a great deal more subtlety than it was on the farm lot, but the idea is the same: somebody wants to be boss. It's not likely that a full-grown adult would say something like, "I'll put up my X-ray Department and dare you to build an Outpatient Surgery Center on top of our parking spaces." But just because the words are not spoken doesn't mean the dare isn't made. There are times when adults feel compelled to wager something they treasure in order to prove their point.

That kind of direct challenge does not happen to most of us very often, but you as a manager should still be prepared for the possibility. Should you accept that kind of challenge to your authority? Here's the rule: Never carry a pocket knife into a gun fight. The winner, and possibly survivor, will be determined on the basis of power. If you don't have the biggest gun, back away. Logic, fairness and being right are probably just pocket knives. Don't engage in those contests unless you're completely sure you cannot lose. Putting up involves honor. It is about your word and your worth to the group. It always involves a personal affront. So if you lose the bet, you lose respect — one of a manager's most precious possessions.

So much for challenges others make. What about challenges *you* make? When should you initiate that kind of dare? Never, if you can help it, because the technique demands that someone lose. You should look for ways for everyone to win. Avoid direct personal challenges, and instead find ways to achieve consensus among people with divergent interests. "Putting up" is almost always destructive, and can almost always be avoided.

Know when to shut up

On the farm lot, the only alternative to putting up was shutting up. That's not the case in management. You don't have to accept every challenge, as we saw in an earlier chapter when a manager simply declared, "I'm not going to put my dog in that fight." Among enlightened adults, the best idea is to make reasonable accommodations so nobody has to lose. Divert personal challenges and keep a dialogue going.

Still, there are times when you should shut up.

Keep in mind that the current topic is "Knowing who is boss." Within that framework, figuring out when to shut up is not very hard: when the boss signals you to keep quiet, do it. The message to shut up takes many forms. A look, a statement, a question, sarcasm, interference or outright anger. However it comes, respect it. Enough said.

A quick, true story: A physician went into partial retirement and was given an important-sounding administrative title so he could continue receiving his full salary. But he apparently didn't realize he wasn't actually supposed to do any administrative work for the money. One day the physician and the administrator locked horns. "You've never had a boss before, have you?" said the physician.

"Sure I have," replied the administrator. "I just didn't know it was you!"

Well, it was.

Here's a pertinent fact of life: as an administrator, arguing with a physician is seriously stupid. You might win a round, but you will never win the fight. Don't even get in the ring. Physicians are the bosses. The title "doctor" is qualification enough. They have the power, even in a case as outrageous as the one above. If you've got to get something done that you know all the physicians won't support, get enough physicians on your side, and let them slug it out among themselves.

In every medical organization there is a group of physicians who think they're the boss. Often they're right; sometimes they're not. But don't assume that just because someone is out of favor at the moment that they'll remain that way. Power comes and goes like the tides. You need to keep track of who's actually in charge at any moment. And if push comes to shove, get out of the way and let opposing factions grind each other down. Be a supply sergeant; give your side whatever support you can, but don't go on the battlefield; you're a non-combatant.

Keep in mind that most medical organizations are like a kitchen with too many cooks. As a medical group manager, you just have to learn to deal with that fact of life. If you can't stand the heat ...

A short diversion here, to say that — amazingly — this book is half over, and the word "Machiavellian" hasn't been used even once. Well, here's the obligatory Machiavellian tip: if you want a decision on a tough issue, put it late on the agenda, and be sure there's at least one meaningless-but-contentious topic to be discussed before it. A true-life example will illustrate:

> Early in an Executive Committee meeting, the chairman (and elder statesman and cagey old fox) said, "Oh, here's something not on the agenda, but give me your thoughts ... Construction on the new office building is ahead of schedule ... Going over some papers, we noticed some of you have specified draperies for your offices and some have asked for venetian blinds. The Design Committee says we need uniformity, so, what do you think it should be? Should we have drapes or blinds?"

Brilliant! *Two hours* of heated discussion followed his question. He didn't rein the discussion in (as he certainly knew how to do when he wanted to), so it ranged all over the place. They literally argued about the kitchen sink. At the end, some members had already left by the time the original agenda items were being dealt with. And one of the last agenda items was an enormously important issue that the chairman didn't want a lot of discussion on — and of course didn't *get* a lot of discussion on, because everyone was already ground down into their socks. Whew! That was a nicely engineered piece of work.

Now, getting back to the topic of "knowing who's boss," keep in mind that in many situations, *you* are the boss. Some of the remaining guidelines take that into consideration.

Know when to keep power

Responsibility and authority must not be given away frivolously. That's the point of this section. Sometimes, for whatever reason, managers delegate things that shouldn't be delegated. This is not as much of a problem as the opposite, when managers try to do everything themselves, but the dangers of over-delegating need to be recognized.

In one way, giving too much power to employees is like giving too much food to guppies; it can actually hurt them. The difference is that overfeeding your fish hurts the fish — not you. But giving away too much power might hurt *you.* Once you've given away power, it's hard to get it back.

Know when to share power with employees

When should you delegate, and when should you refrain from it? The guiding principle is this: delegate a task to an employee only when you are pretty confident it will get done properly, and when you'd be willing to part with it permanently if you had to, *and* when you are trying to groom the employee for greater responsibility.

Lots of things fit these criteria. Lots of things don't. You must be the one to decide between them.

Empowering employees is a very good idea — if they understand the agenda, will stick to it, and will be accountable for performance. Empower employees who do those things; keep power away from employees who don't do those things.

How can you tell which ones will, and which ones won't? You observe and you analyze.

Let's say your clinic has decided that Dr. Godley is right: it's important to get the physician, the patient and the medical record in the room at the same time. This is supposed to be on everyone's "to do" list; it's supposed to be on everyone's agenda. Is it? How do you tell? Watch employees in action. What do they consistently do? Listen to their words. What do they consistently discuss? Notice their emotional investment. What feelings operate in their work and relationships? The answers will determine which employees are candidates for greater responsibility.

So far this chapter has concentrated on the relationship between bosses and the people who work for them. But in most work settings, the majority of relationships are officially peer-to-peer. That leads to the next guideline.

Know how to share power with peers

Let's strain the breathing analogy a bit. No one person can breathe all the air, and no one person can exercise all the power. Managers have to breathe the common air of power in the organization. As managers we must take care of our specific responsibilities, while always being conscious of the good of the organization as a whole.

Managers normally share power with each other by discussing common concerns, because actions in one area may impact every other area. When Medicare changes its rules about the use of Unique Provider Numbers on claims forms, for example, the Data Processing Department will bear most of the burden of the new regulations. But if that department didn't respond properly, claims would be denied, money would stop flowing, and eventually all the departments would suffer. So everyone needs to be involved to some extent.

Discussions among managers occur without hard and fast rules for the working relationships. The organization chart doesn't often help. Here's a good, practical rule for sharing power with peers: when working on an issue in another person's area, think of yourself as a trusted employee working for that person. And when peers are working in your area, they should do the same for you. This approach recognizes that one person occupies a "first among equals" position on the particular issue at hand. It demonstrates an ability to cooperate in difficult circumstances. It indicates the desire to focus on the good of the organization. And it saves the energy that combat would require.

But of course every organization has human "lawnmowers" who cut up everything in sight. They typically attempt to build their power at the expense of others. They feel tall only when they cut someone else down. Here's a rule for sharing power with peers when mutual respect and cooperation are difficult: don't play the game. It's that simple. Let them do what they will. Do what you need to do. If they act outside their permissions, the persons with the real power will take care of them. Relax, approach it as a student and learn about power.

Sharing power with peers requires walking a narrow line. On the one hand, managers must cooperate with each other. On the other hand, some people can be overbearing and unfair. There's no need for you to be a doormat. Here is one final rule that applies when the games can't be avoided: Don't try to win; instead, try not to lose.

The 100 percent effective method not to lose at tennis: always manage to hit the ball back across the net. Just dink it across. Don't try to slam it. Don't try to finesse the other person. See the point? If you can't avoid the game, just keep hitting the ball back into the other person's court.

Those who start games look for a payoff. You provide it by playing their game on their terms — they become boss. But if you can manage to hit the ball back to them endlessly, you'll deprive them of their payoff. They'll quit in frustration.

There's one more guideline, and it is enormously important.

Count your votes

A lot of business decisions are voted on. Not formally in meetings, but informally, every day. Most people have learned to ask the opinion of other people on issues that might be controversial; most people are gregarious, and look for consensus where they can. So in the day-to-day exchanges, a lot of ideas are proposed, a lot of opinions are expressed and a lot of voting is done.

This kind of voting occurs without anyone ever saying the word "vote." When the medical records supervisor says, "Do you think the chart labels should be white or tan?" your response is going to be tallied as a vote. If the lab director asks you whether you think the clinic needs a new immunoassay machine, you're being polled.

Knowing who's boss on a particular issue is often a matter of knowing how many votes someone has. The easy part is the counting. The hard part is counting *accurately*. But it is essential to count votes.

Many important decisions are made in meetings. Here's some essential advice: don't ever go into a meeting unless you know what's going to happen there. Otherwise you might get blind-sided. Know what the agenda is, know what's going to be voted on and know how the vote will go.

Impossible? Not really, but it takes practice. If you think it is impossible to know in advance what's going to happen at a meeting, watch closely how powerful individuals in your organization behave at meetings. See if they act like anything is a surprise to them. No? That's because nothing *is* a surprise. They already know everything that's going to happen. They learned this lesson a long time ago. Counting your votes is a lot easier if the votes are in your pocket.

A lot of decisions are made in meetings, but without an actual vote. There will be some discussion, a general buzz of acclamation, and the next topic will be introduced. (Just in case you've wondered, yes it is true in medicine that if there are six people at a meeting, there will be eight opinions expressed on any issue: two of the people will change their minds by the time the discussion gets back around to them.)

Here's a war story about counting votes.

Gail was the data processing manager at the regional office of a major pharmaceutical company. She ran a tight ship and ran it with an iron fist. She was ambitious, tough and hard-working; she was accustomed to getting what she wanted.

Sherri was at the same level in the company. She was in charge of sales of OTC medications to hospitals in the region — a big, important job. She ran a tight ship, and didn't put up with any nonsense — but was known to be generous and supportive with her employees. She, too, was ambitious, tough and hard-working; and she was accustomed to getting what she wanted — but what she wanted was usually what her team agreed was best. She worked through consensus rather than mandate.

Are we about to see a fight between good and evil? No. But the stage certainly has been set for a drama demonstrating the importance of counting your votes, and a conflict involving two different approaches to the use of power. Gail and Sherri's company had selected their region as the test market for a new line of non-aspirin pain killers. Sherri had been asked to manage the hospital part of the roll-out, which included a big marketing push in drugstores and physicians' offices. This was going to be a big deal.

The overall plan had been introduced at a big meeting of executive staff and managers. After that, managers were expected to meet individually or in groups, as needed, to define the details and the effects on their departments. Then there would be another big meeting to see where things stood.

Sherri met with Gail to get ideas on inventory control and order processing from a data processing perspective and to get the names of the data processing employees assigned to work with Sherri and her department. Gail gave her lots of ideas, a great many of which were far beyond Gail's area of responsibility — which didn't stop her from insisting that they be implemented. Sherri listened, thanked Gail for her ideas, and said she would take them into account. Sherri also indicated that she viewed some of the issues differently, particularly the inventory control.

Gail's department really wouldn't be affected much by all this, since most of the needed systems were already in place. But Gail tried to stake a claim on any future rewards, saying she expected to be extensively involved, "to avoid a data processing catastrophe." She was repeating the behaviors that had extended her control far beyond her place on the organization chart. Why could she do it? She had the gold, a title that included the words "data processing."

Most managers would not go to the trouble of understanding the automated systems, so they had to go to her with hat in hand for help. Her price for helping was control.

Sherri did go to the trouble of understanding the automated systems. She outlined the inventory operations based on her thoughts and based on Gail's ideas. Gail had some pretty good ideas and Sherri incorporated them. However, Gail's need for control would build in unneeded steps and would require Sherri's employees to continually line up outside Gail's office waiting for information they needed.

Sherri met with each of the other managers and talked them through her operations design. She incorporated their suggestions and asked for any additional ideas. She followed up with memoranda verifying the revised design. Then she met with the designated people in the Data Processing Department to verify and document the capabilities and limitations of the automated system. In all this she was doing her job — and she was gathering votes. She sent a draft of a management summary to the CEO and got it back with his approval. Then she sent it to the other managers, including Gail. The summary enraged Gail. She called Sherri and said, "I just want you to know that I am going to the CEO and tell him I think you are going about this all wrong."

"Well, he is the CEO, and if he wants to make some changes, that's fine with me," was Sherri's reply. There was no further communication from Gail. The big internal meeting came and went without a hitch and the new product hit the market successfully. Everyone received praise from the CEO and he made a special point to compliment the Data Processing Department on the smoothness with which they undertook the implementation.

Let's make some observations from this story. First, Sherri counted her votes. She knew exactly who her supporters were because she gave them reasons in terms of their self-interest to endorse her ideas. Second, she refused to enter a power struggle with Gail. She did what was right for the company, the customers and the employees. Third, Gail had assumed that Sherri would follow her suggestions, even after Sherri outlined areas of difference. Gail's assumption allowed Sherri to control the timing and packaging of the unavoidable confrontation. Fourth, counting votes is not the secret of success: *getting* votes is. Sherri got support. Each of the managers had input into the process, and had the information to plan their operations and train their people far in advance; it was easy for them to go along with Sherri.

Notice that the only loser was the person who tried to make a win/lose situation of the issue in the first place — Gail. She lost only in her mind. The CEO thought she and her people had done a brilliant job. The other managers felt better about data processing now than ever before. But Gail felt like a loser and acted like a loser. Her need for control was so great that she could see the issue in no other terms. Sherri had an enemy as long as both of them stayed in the same organization.

People do things like that. That is why it is necessary to count your votes. In order to do what's right, managers must often engage in such politics. Gail felt Sherri had undermined her. In fact, Sherri had simply decided not to lose. That is different from winning. Sherri carefully avoided every win/lose element. She carefully made all recommendations so nobody had to lose — unless they insisted, as Gail did. But Sherri did not expect Gail to understand. She was not disappointed: those who operate with a win/lose mentality do not understand the distinction between "winning" and "not losing."

Knowing who is boss is knowing about power. We are avoiding the temptation to talk about how power *should* be exercised in order to talk about how it is *actually* exercised. Knowing who is boss is the key to getting things done and avoiding damage to your career.

So, wait a minute, all this power stuff does not sound like fun. Why can't I just do my job and not worry about power? Because that is not the way the world works. Simply choosing strawberry yogurt instead of peach ice cream is an exercise of power. Merely asking a question exercises power — the power to question or define the agenda. Remember the breathing analogy. People breathe continuously and without any conscious intervention in the process. We and those around us in the work place exercise power continuously and we should pay great attention to it.

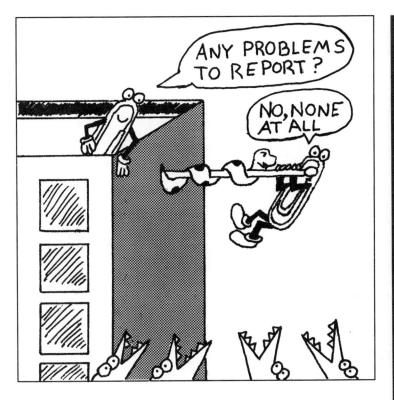

Report
problems
and
ask for help

Among linguists there's an old story about a Scotsman who fell into a lake. A group of Englishmen on the shore watched in respectful silence as the Scotsman, bobbing up and down, shouted, "I will drown, and no one shall help me!"

That's the whole story. To understand it you need to know that Scotsmen and Englishmen sometimes use the words "will" and "shall" oppositely. When the Scotsman yelled, "I will drown, and no one shall help me," he meant, "I am about to drown, and no one intends to help me." But the Englishmen on the shore interpreted his words to mean, "I intend to drown, and no one should help me!" They didn't interfere because they thought the Scotsman wanted to commit suicide!

Pointy-headed intellectuals love that story. The rest of us intellectuals might manage a thin smile once the story is explained to us. Still, we chose to use it here to make a point: even if you want to report problems and ask for help (as the drowning man certainly did), sometimes it is harder than you think it will be. So in this chapter we will discuss both the benefits and the difficulties of reporting problems and asking for help. In other words, we'll cover both the "why" and the "how."

Create an official policy for fouling up and reporting problems

Here's something to think about: What is the official policy for screwing up in your organization? What? You don't have one? Wow, where did you find all these great employees who don't need an official way to report problems and ask for help?

One of the authors loves to begin seminars with those questions. The answers are predictable, usually including, "Fire the person who screwed up," "Pray," and "Hope no one finds out." This last response leads to another question. "What if you make a really bad mistake, but no one knows about it and it will probably remain unknown for several months. In an ideal world, how would you like to handle it?" The answer is equally predictable. Most people say, "I would like to be able to tell my boss without being treated like an idiot, being yelled at or being threatened with the loss of my job."

Everybody fouls up. That's human nature. Some people do it regularly. Sometimes there are heavy consequences. That's life. Most people cover up their mistakes because organizations reward cover-ups instead of rewarding candor. Many organizations also punish employees for asking for help, using this logic: "If you need help, we made a mistake placing you in the position."

Would organizations benefit by making it safe to admit mistakes? Yes. Making mistakes and needing help are not character disorders. Therefore, we suggest developing and publishing a policy for screwing up and asking for help. The policy might look something like this:

Official policy for screwing up and asking for help

The Generic Clinic recognizes that no employee is perfect. Therefore, employees who make honest mistakes in the absence of clear instructions are encouraged to report them immediately. There will be no adverse consequences for employees who immediately report honest mistakes, unless legal or other outside standards require action against the employee.

> Further, The Generic Clinic recognizes that even the most qualified employee does not know everything. Therefore, employees are encouraged to ask for help to gain the knowledge and skills to perform their jobs, when needed. There will be no adverse consequences to employees who ask for this help.
>
> On the other hand, there *will be* adverse consequences for employees who do not report mistakes that are found later, and there *will be* adverse consequences for employees who do not ask for help when needed. Reporting problems and asking for help will be treated as a development opportunity.

What a concept! Make it easy for employees to manage their lack of perfection.

What about you as a manager, as a person who has to decide what to tell and what to hide from your superiors. Should you make it a practice to report problems and ask for help? Yes. Why? Because it can save your hide, that's why. But many medical group managers have trouble putting this axiom into practice. The concept sometimes seems contrary to two natural laws.

The first natural law is: *people hide problems.* The second one is: *in a crunch, people want to do it themselves.*

People hide problems

You don't believe it? Remember Jonathan, the farmer's son? One day when he was about 12 years old, Jonathan was showing off to some of his buddies, taking them joy riding on his dad's tractor. Jonathan knew how to drive the tractor, but in his effort to impress his friends he drove too fast down a hill. At the bottom of the hill the road made a 90° turn and ran parallel to a woven wire fence. At the bottom of the hill Jonathan made an 80° turn, ran into the fence, got a wheel tangled up in the wire, and tore out about 40 feet of fine fencing. He came to rest in a cornfield, after scaring the life out of a sow and eight pigs.

Jonathan shut off the engine and looked around for his buddies, but of course they had all jumped off and had run for home. He went back to the house, got the wirecutters, cut the fence loose from the tractor and put the tractor back in the shed. He acted like nothing happened. Nervously, he acted calm.

It is not hard to guess that his father discovered the downed fence, the damaged cornfield and the newly-liberated pigs. Nor is it hard to guess that he figured Jonathan probably had something to do with it.

It is easy to dismiss Jonathan's effort to hide the problem as the behavior of an immature child. But how do you explain the behavior of a 35-year-old finance manager who learned her agency was going to be hit hard with an audit, but — true story — decided not to report it because she knew she'd have to postpone vacation to deal with it. Immaturity?

In reality, this type of behavior is not uncommon. People try to keep superiors from knowing that something has gone wrong.

Why is it that some lessons of childhood are easily remembered and some are not? Jonathan's dad found out the truth — as parents nearly always do. The finance manager's superiors found out about the audit — as they were bound to do. Sheesh! Why is our impulse to hide things so strong — particularly when it is so unlikely those things will stay hidden?

Not only that, but when the truth is revealed, the boss/parent/ spouse/friend/patient/customer has every reason to be angry about it. It's a double whammy: not only do you have a problem to deal with, but you also have someone angry with you. We hope to show you later that life doesn't have to be like that.

In a crunch, people want to do it themselves

The second natural law that this axiom seems to contradict is this: in a crunch people want to do it themselves. Or at least they don't want anybody else to do it. We have a story about Jonathan's father that illustrates this.

Jonathan and his parents were going south to sunny Florida one winter. Jonathan's father really got white-knuckled whenever he drove in heavy traffic or on unfamiliar roads, and he hated driving in the mountains. The best route from the farm to the beach was over the top of a very big mountain near Chattanooga, Tennessee. Now this vacation took place in the days before the interstate highways were completed, so the family realized that all the conditions the dad hated most were lying in wait for them in the great state of Tennessee.

They decided to drive around the mountain. Obviously this was a longer route, but the family all agreed to it.

The alternate route took them west of Chattanooga through northern Alabama to Phoenix City, where they would cross the border into Columbus, Georgia. Leaving Phoenix City, Jonathan pointed out to his father that they hadn't crossed a river (which the map showed), they hadn't seen another town (Columbus), and they hadn't seen a sign saying, "Welcome to Georgia!"

Jonathan's father didn't believe in constructive criticism and he didn't want a child correcting him. Jonathan's mother stayed out of the argument so she could later join whoever had been right in saying, "We knew you were wrong all along," to the one who had been mistaken. (Do you know someone in your organization who takes this approach?)

They were verging on dysfunctional family behavior, of course, but remember this was a long time ago — there were no experts or self-help books to tell them that they were dysfunctional, so they thought their behavior was pretty normal.

Jonathan kept saying, "Why don't you stop and ask somebody?" His Dad kept driving south insisting that he was in Georgia. Finally — either to shut Jonathan up or because he was beginning to have doubts himself — the dad stopped at a service station to inquire about where they were.

The attendant said in a heavy southern accent, "Dothan."

"Dawson?" the Dad responded.

"No, Dothan," came the reply.

"Dothan, Georgia?" asked the Dad.

"No, Dothan, Alabama," replied the attendant.

Not to belabor the point, but they were pretty far off course. In fact they were within 20 miles of the Florida border, but about 200 miles west of where they should have been. All because Jonathan's dad did not want to ask for help. In the crunch, he wanted to do everything himself.

When you suspect your organization has taken a wrong turn, pipe up! If you see a problem, don't keep it a secret, even if you caused it. *Especially* if you caused it. Ask for help. Don't try to go it alone. If you take this axiom to heart, you'll be amazed at the difference it makes. Sure you'll still have the original problem to deal with, but instead of people being angry with you, most of the time they'll be supportive and sympathetic. So fess up. You'll be glad you did. It will save you a ton of embarrassed backpedaling.

If you don't tell those who need to know, they'll find out anyway

Again, if you don't tell people who need to know, they'll find out anyway. They always do. And if you struggle to do everything yourself, the people who ought to know will find that out, too. They will either hear rumors or someone will try to make points at your expense by telling them.

It's bad enough when you don't inform your employees of something they need to know, but it's even worse to keep your boss in the dark. If the boss comes to you and says, "What's this I hear about such-and-so?" you are two notches behind already. You're a boss, right? And you don't like being kept in the dark, right? Nobody does — including your employees, and even more so, your boss.

How to report problems and ask for help

Remember the axiom "Timing is almost everything" in deciding when to expose a problem. You must find the right moment, but you mustn't wait too long. You can't hide a problem forever. All things being equal, if it's something in your area of responsibility, the best strategy is to make sure the boss and everyone else knows about it as soon as possible. If your boss hears about it from someone else, you may lose control and you will probably lose respect.

An administrator of a small group practice was having computer problems. Nothing he did for hours and hours seemed to work. Finally about 4 p.m. he had it working properly. Being sure of his success he told all the physicians that it was fixed and everything would be okay the next day.

But then he found another problem. He stayed at the office frantically trying to solve it, but again nothing seemed to work. He called a service bureau but they were closed. He called a friend who said, "Gosh, you've got a serious problem. (pause) Good luck." He finally realized that no one was available to help him at this late hour and that he couldn't do it himself.

Exhausted, he went home at 11:30 p.m. He slept fitfully for a few hours and dreamed about the chaos that would take place the next morning when the physicians arrived to find that the appointment system still was not working.

He went back to the office at 7 a.m. and started again. He didn't tell the physicians that his announcement the previous day had been premature and that the office was still a mess. One by one they came in and discovered the problem, and — depending on their personality type (remember "different strokes for different folks") — they reacted either negatively or *really* negatively.

Needless to say, no one nominated this administrator for an MGMA award that year. He survived in his job because otherwise he was a pretty competent manager, but he learned a valuable lesson.

Stay calm

When it is time to tell people about a problem, also remember the axiom about "packaging." Don't run around the office wringing your hands and saying, "Oh, we have a *problem!*" Instead be calm, and give a simple explanation. Use simple, direct and unequivocal statements. Don't end up like the hapless Scotsman at the beginning of the chapter: Be sure you are speaking the same language as the people you are addressing.

Give an accurate account of the problem

Don't gloss over important issues, and don't paint a rosy picture. In fact, you are probably better off to present the darkest picture you can accurately paint. That way you won't understate the challenge being faced, and (as a side benefit) your eventual accomplishments will be measured against the *perceived* threat. Offer solutions if you can, and try to make your definition of "success" fit the image of success as seen by the others who will be affected — particularly your superiors.

Don't overpromise

If a department, such as Medical Records, has been marginal for a long time and has finally ground to a halt, don't promise that soon you'll have it running perfectly. It took a long time for it to stop and it will take some time for it to get going again. And some things will never be fixed. For example, if the documentation in your medical records is bad, the best you can do is to *begin* to document things properly. You can't undo the past. You can't "fix" the problem of poor records from previous years; you can only start today to eliminate the problem from this day forward.

Be prepared

If you work directly with physicians, there's something you should know: When you make a mistake, the physicians' first instinct will be to fire you. It's not the physicians' fault they're like that. They are trained to be like that. Physicians are trained to identify what's "wrong," and to find what's causing it. They're professional faultfinders and they practice their craft every day. In their field they are rewarded for making quick and accurate diagnoses based on sketchy information, then identifying root causes, and then — here's the good part — attacking the cause, with the fervent desire and the zealous professional intention of killing it dead, dead, dead.

Like generals, physicians do battle — against disease and discomfort and disfigurement. They zap cells with radiation, they obliterate bacteria with deadly chemicals, they vaporize tissue with lasers, they remove, alter, implant, inject, debride, defibrillate. They slash and burn, they suture and salve. The body is the battlefield and the enemy is a diseased organ, a clump of malformed tissue or a platoon of wayward cells.

Or, the enemy can be an entire person. Somebody like you, or one of your employees. Somebody who has done something "wrong." How do you think a physician is going to regard the luckless clerk who triple-books an appointment slot? Like a close friend? Ha! In the physician's eyes at that moment, that employee has begun taking on the appearance of a cancer cell.

When physicians see an administrative problem, they sometimes propose solutions that will work — in isolation and at the expense of some other aspect of the operation. ("Yes, Doctor," you hear yourself saying, "firing Janet *will* keep her from ever overbooking your appointment slots again.") And unfortunately, the way medical organizations are inevitably organized, the physicians don't have only medical responsibilities: they are also given final oversight responsibilities for administration — the one area where their training and often their interest is notoriously lacking.

So give them some slack; it's not their fault they act that way.

But this book isn't about physicians, it's about managers. And the point in this chapter is that as a manager you will often have to report problems to physicians, the physicians won't be at all grateful for the news, and the physicians will want to fire you. No, what they really want is to give you a brain transplant — and THEN fire you.

Time for the Boy Scout's motto. Whenever you must report administrative problems to physicians, "Be prepared."

Give the physicians (and anyone else involved) all the information you have in a calm, confident manner. You want them to understand the nature of the problem and to feel like you know what you are doing. You want them to be supportive, but you don't want the boss to send in someone else to handle the situation because it looks too big for you to handle yourself. When bosses start taking over and solving your problems, they have a legitimate right to wonder why you should survive the next budget crisis.

Put it into practice

While working on this book, one of the authors had a problem like the computer foul-up described above, except that this was a phone system problem. It all started routinely enough: The practice had grown and needed several new phones added to the system. He thought briefly about doing the work himself to save money and time, but wisely decided to call in the experts: in a medical practice, telecommunications are critical, and are simply too important to take chances with. So, at 4:30 p.m., incoming calls were forwarded to the answering service, and the experts arrived.

They came, they saw, they screwed up.

To make a long story short, everything was haywire for about a week. Every fix failed, and instead of having an expanded system, a dozen phones had to be disconnected to keep the system working at all. Limping along with half a phone system was a chore, but — remembering the axiom "report problems" and remembering the story of the computer system fiasco — the author was careful to keep the physicians and department supervisors closely informed about what was happening.

It worked beautifully. Everyone worked as a team. Instead of complaining, everyone accepted the challenge, and worked hard to get through a difficult period. What could have been an administrative disaster turned into an opportunity for the team to shine, and the difficulties were taken in stride.

Anticipate "opportunities"

Now, a tough question: What if you work in a place where mistakes are not tolerated? What if the bosses make it clear that they don't want to hear your problems, and that they regard problems as mistakes and mistakes as failures?

Here's some good advice: Find another job. Oh, you want practical advice. Okay: Find another job.

But if that excellent advice won't work for you, here's what you have to do. You have to work really hard at anticipating problems, so you can present them as "concerns" or as "opportunities," not problems. And you must do this long, long, *long* before they turn into real problems that need immediate attention. And you must make your concerns public, at least to the extent that they are documented in an agenda or a memo, so you don't end up being the sacrificial lamb.

"Has anybody noticed any over-bookings, or anything else unusual about scheduling?" you can say at the monthly meeting. "Can anyone think of ways we might improve the system?" Then keep quiet. Mention the need for additional staff training (or whatever else you need to avoid a catastrophe) only if nobody else mentions it. There. Now you've raised the issue, and you've started the process for making positive changes, and the whole thing is "on record" in the minutes of the meeting. Good job.

What about recognition for getting that job done? Who's going to praise you for steering around land mines that other people didn't even realize were there? Forget it. Sometimes you just have to hide your light under a basket. Showing how bright you are won't win you any friends among people who want to be left in the dark.

Be careful

Okay, next variation. In an environment where problems are not tolerated, what do you do about big problems that come up completely without warning, and that you did not anticipate?

The best thing you can do is keep your résumé current.

Really, this is a tough question. The answer is you can duck, and hope the bullets don't find you, or you can stand tall and hope the bullets bounce off. If you are a superperson, you have nothing to worry about. If you're mortal, scurry around like everyone else, covering your tracks.

Judge carefully and learn to wait

Next topic: What if the problem you want to report doesn't belong to you? Who do you tell? When? How? It depends! You have to be careful when you are trying to expose a problem that is not in your area of responsibility. Be careful how you offer help or reveal the problem. If you run in too quickly and talk about someone else, you are seen as a backstabber. If you wait until catastrophe occurs and the boss figures out that you saw it coming and didn't do anything, your loyalty might justifiably be called into question.

This really is an area that calls for careful judgment. The first chapter of this book says sometimes you must wait to present your ideas until enough pain has been endured by those who might benefit from them. True. But allowing some anticipatory discomfort is different from allowing a catastrophe.

Just as you want your own boss to be supportive without being intrusive, it is important for you to know when to stand by and let your people take their own shot at getting a job done. Sometimes you literally have to stand there with your arms folded, waiting. Waiting is scary, but it works.

One of the authors once planned and coordinated a state-wide conference for 300 elderly citizens. He delegated transportation, an important and challenging task, to a member of his staff.

There was a big session in an auditorium, after which the participants were supposed to board shuttle buses back to their individual dormitories. Each dorm had a specific bus assigned to it. In other words, if you got on the wrong bus, you'd end up at the wrong dorm.

When the session was over the participants crowded into the lobby. There was a heavy rain coming down outside. The buses were all lined up in the street. Looking at the buses from the lobby, through the rain, the participants couldn't readily tell which bus they were supposed to get on: the buses all looked the same.

The author saw the crowd of people milling around in the lobby and felt he should do something. Something like, you know, taking charge. But he didn't know, any better than anyone else, which bus was going where. And the staff person responsible for transportation, the person who did know the shuttle assignments, was nowhere to be seen.

He waited for an eternity, resisting the temptation to do something, until she arrived. Sure enough, she rushed in and promptly brought order to what could have turned into something like the evacuation of Saigon.

So at times you should literally fold your arms and watch. Most managers don't do this often enough. A supervisor walks through a clinic and hears a telephone ringing, or sees patients backed up. Instead of thinking calmly about what is wrong and who should be taking care of it, the supervisor picks up the phone and starts scheduling appointments. When the crunch is over, the supervisor continues down the hall.

But the next time there is an overload the same thing happens. Some supervisors spend too much time actually *doing* things, and they don't think about why the problems are happening and how to eliminate them. The employees know that the supervisor will bail them out, so some employees take advantage of the situation. They never worry about getting behind — they just let the supervisor pitch in, day after day.

One reason supervisors need to delegate tasks to others is so the supervisors can spend more time worrying about how to avoid problems — and less time dealing with today's brush fires. If you want a quick litmus test for the ability to delegate, ask the supervisors who work for you to "fold their arms and watch." One administrator we know tried this with a supervisor. The supervisor was unable to do it and suffered a great deal for it. Whenever she saw something wrong, her need to fix it herself was so great that, ultimately, she and the administrator agreed she wasn't cut out to be a supervisor.

You must get your people involved, and not do everything yourself. You must give them the time and resources to get it done.

Communicate to employees and supervisors

Everybody working in a medical group has to see themselves as being in the same boat. Everybody has an oar and everybody should be rowing in the same direction. The goal may be simply to keep the boat from sinking, it may be to get to shore, it may be to get to shore within a certain period of time, but everybody in the boat has to be part of the same effort. Otherwise, you could be paddling in circles.

The axiom "Report problems and ask for help" is actually a part of the larger issue of effective communication. When everyone is in the same boat, everyone needs to know what's going on — but most especially when there are problems.

Who is on your list of people to ask for help? It should contain everyone, up and down the line.

Ask your boss

Remember the axiom that says, "You never have a problem, only an opportunity." Think "opportunity" when you ask your boss for help. Solving the immediate problem is a given; what else might you accomplish? It may be an opportunity to get resources you wanted earlier but couldn't justify. Ask for everything you need to solve the problem, but don't be greedy.

Ask your employees

As you go about solving problems, give your people the time and resources to do the actual work. Let them fix problems. Whatever is broken, they probably had something to do with breaking it in the first place, didn't they? So don't just wade in and fix it yourself. Meet with your key people, listen to their ideas and opinions, tell them what you expect and, if it is appropriate, fold your arms and watch.

Let them help you. Push the work to them. Push the decision making to them. Watch them, monitor them and have checkpoints along the way. When there is no crisis, your checkpoints may be less frequent. When you are facing a crisis your checkpoints may be daily to let people know you are monitoring progress, but the idea is still to make them the owners of the problem and let them fix it.

Ask your peers

All medical group managers have the same problems. Most are willing to share ideas and helpful hints with others. People will help you if they see you as likable and as someone who in turn will help them. Your problems have been faced by others before you. Don't be shy. Pick up the phone and call. Medical Group Management Association provides excellent peer resources through its membership.

Ask your friends

You may be surprised to learn that your friends in other lines of work can often relate to your problems. We know a consultant who had two major clients at the same time — one was a sheet metal fabricator; the other, a medical clinic. He swears that the problems were the same and to a great extent so were the solutions.

Final thoughts

It's a simple axiom, "Report problems and ask for help." It only defies two natural laws. Ask yourself every day if there is something you need to report or something you need help with. If the answer is yes (the answer is always yes), then ask, "Who do I need to tell? When? How? Whose help do I need?"

Train your employees to do the same. Teach them that it's human to foul things up. Tell them: "If you mess up, fess up." Teach them to ask for help.

If you practice this axiom you have a better than fighting chance to keep your backside intact.

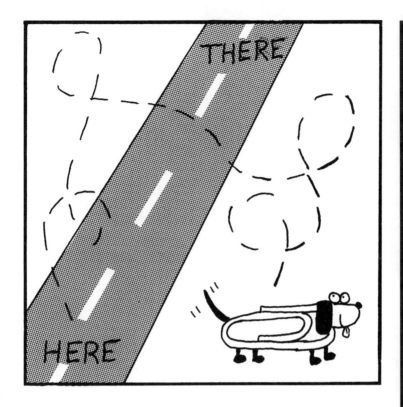

AXIOM 8

Plan what you do and do what you plan

J onathan's six-month-old beagle pup, Ed, discovered his hunting instinct one morning. Jonathan watched Ed leave the dog house and run hard down an interesting rabbit trail, his nose to the ground and his tail wagging. Both the boy and the pup were smiling in delight.

Many people don't know it, but even pure-bred hunting dogs must be taught to hunt if they're going to reach their potential. "Not every dog learns to hunt on its own," thought Jonathan, proudly. His pride faded as he checked on Ed's progress. Ed never followed a trail very far. He stopped, looked around, smelled the ground and the air in several directions, frowned in indecision and with a "what the heck" wave of this tail, took off on a new direction until he crossed another trail.

Ed managed to cram a hundred acres of hunting into a ten acre field and never did see a rabbit. "That dumb dog can't hunt," Jonathan said to his dad when Ed staggered home footsore and hungry. His father was more understanding, saying, "Sure he can hunt. He just wasn't hunting anything in particular. And that's what he found." The dad let that notion sink in for a moment, and then added a final thought: "Maybe you ought to teach him to hunt."

The authors know a manager who acts like Ed the Beagle. No one is busier, no one more intense. Ed the Manager rushes to meetings, he arrives late for appointments and he misses some events and activities altogether. With very little prompting he'll recite for you his list of problems that are out of control and projects that are

107

behind schedule. It is a common sight in Ed's department to see haggard employees stalking in the hallways like hungry mountain lions, looking for Ed, so they can get his signature on this-or-that document needed to meet this-or-that deadline. Ed is always on the run, shirt tail flying in the wind, trailing a string of problems. He stumbles to his office at the end of the day, tired and hungry, never having seen the management rabbit.

Ed the Beagle and Ed the Manager are our case for the importance of Axiom 8: Plan what you do and do what you plan.

Lacking training, both Ed the Beagle and Ed the Manager do their jobs instinctively, as best they know how. Likewise, Ed the Manager's employees do their jobs instinctively. It would make a difference for all of these creatures if their bosses would take time to teach them the basics of planning. The basics are to understand the goal and then to figure out how you intend to reach it, before you actually begin heading that way. If you can do just that much, you'll avoid going down a lot of false trails.

So the point of "Plan what you do and do what you plan" is to outline how to achieve success — after first answering the critical question, "What does success look like?"

As we saw in an earlier chapter, bosses are responsible for answering that question. If you're the boss of a hunting dog, you ought to have a clear mental picture of what a hard day on the trails will produce. If you're the boss of a department, clinic or a hospital, you ought to have a clear mental picture of what a hard day's work will produce. You can't be a good and effective boss if you can't picture success and communicate that picture to the people who work for you.

There's nothing scary or mysterious about planning. Many people do a terrific job of it when they plan their vacations. They get maps, guidebooks, brochures, rate sheets, calendars and schedules — *data*. They spread all this stuff out on a table, read it, and say things like, "No, if we stay in Orlando through Friday night, we can't make it to New Orleans in time for the parade on Saturday. So we have to leave Orlando on Friday morning at the latest." In other words, they decide what it is they want to do, and then they figure out how to do it.

That's the "plan what you do" part of this axiom. The "do what you plan" part, in this case, happens when the happy vacationers get in the car or on the plane, and go out and have a heck of a good time. Right? You bet. Easy? You bet.

So we can do the same thing at work, right? Get the data, study it, decide on some stuff and hit the bricks. Right?

Yes! And no! The fundamental precepts are the same for vacation planning and for operational planning at work, yet most people do a better job applying Axiom 8 to vacations than they do applying it to work.

Obstacles to planning

Why is business planning harder? For one thing, most people lack training, experience and encouragement. But there's a more significant reason, and it is this: in business you are almost always shooting at a moving target.

That's not the case with vacations: Orlando is still where it was last year, and the road that used to go to New Orleans, we can say with assurance, still goes right to New Orleans. There's a lot you can count on when planning a vacation, a lot of *certainty*. But with business there's an enormous amount of *uncertainty* that has to be dealt with.

Competition

What kinds of uncertainty? Well, for instance, uncertainty about what the competition will do.

To expand the vacation analogy a bit, pretend you had to deal with competition on vacation. Not just other vacationers who might get ahead of you in the ticket line. Oh, no, we mean COMPETITION — hard-hearted people who hate your guts, and who *seriously* want you out of the picture. If you let 'em, they'll steal your car keys, or put sand in your gas tank. They'll put up phony road signs to confuse you. They'll pass you doing 90 and throw tacks out their windows. They'll blow up bridges. Hey, these people want to *EAT YOUR LUNCH.*

Well, that would certainly make vacation planning a bit more intense, wouldn't it?

Competition in medicine differs in some respects from competition in the world of commerce, but don't kid yourself by thinking it does not exist, or that it does not matter. For every bankrupt HMO, there is a now-broken network of providers who can attest to the effects of competition. Keep in mind that these providers were in the business of medicine, not the business of insurance. Tough luck: the bullet of competition killed the HMO, and it wounded everyone else in the network. You see the point.

The changing marketplace

This plays havoc with business planning. Customers' habits and tastes change: This year it's *Buy American*, next year it's *Why pay more?* One year it's *Luxury at affordable prices*, the next year it's *Luxury at luxury prices*. Some goods go from *Cheap at twice the price* to *Cheap at half the price* in one season.

Medicine doesn't suffer so much from these wild and woolly market swings, but at the same time, medicine is not immune to them. For example, the numbers are sharply declining for hysterectomies, Cesarean deliveries and screening chest X-rays, because (to some extent) of a changing marketplace. Another example: as the population ages, gerontologists will come into their own, and specialists such as sports medicine physicians may see business decline. All these things affect revenues and jobs.

The government

Another uncertainty, particularly in medicine, is what the government has up its sleeve. For instance, when the federal government's intentions are unclear on the issue of "PPR" (Physician Payment Reform), how can medical organizations plan long-term expansions? How are your plans (and your ability to plan) affected when state legislators threaten to set fees for health care services?

Research and technology

Another factor that makes business planning much more difficult than vacation planning is the march of research and technology. This is especially true in medicine. Ask urologists whether blasting kidney stones with lithotripsy has changed the way they practice. Ask dentists, whose revenue from filling cavities, dropped out of sight in one generation after fluoridation. Ask a polio expert about technology — if you can find one. Their practices changed dramatically and in a short time after effective vaccines were discovered.

Not that anyone would wish anything else, but from a planning perspective one must ask the question: What are oncologists going to do if someone finds a cure for cancer?

You can see the point. Technology is a two-edged sword. One year a manufacturing plant turns out ten million vinyl record albums, the next year the plant is out of business as the plant down the street produces ten million compact disks. When you are planning your vacation there is not really a "technology" factor to worry about, but in business it can be enormously important.

Changing values

Another uncertainty that affects business planning is the future value of money. Another (and this one can reach way down within any organization, medical or otherwise) is the changing of the guard: people retire and things change.

How to plan

So, as managers, how do we deal with this? First, we count our blessings. Second, we *continually* plan what we do and do what we plan; we *continually* re-define what the goals are and what it takes to succeed, and we *continually* pay a lot more attention to business planning than we do to vacation planning — because it's a lot trickier. Planning what you do and doing what you plan is a way to provide structure for managing in uncertain times.

Count your blessings

Why does it say up there that the first thing we do is count our blessings? Because the very uncertainty that makes planning tricky is what creates jobs for managers. Without that uncertainty, organizations could operate with a clerical staff. One manager says: "While I like 'no brainers,' people who do them day in and day out end up with no brains." Uncertainty provides job security and the challenge that fuels managerial growth.

And while we're counting our blessings, let's get some perspective. If you're a manager (and not something like a Senior Supreme High Executive Presidential Administrator) you're not among those in your organization who have to worry about the really enormous questions of technology and changing marketplaces and competition. In military terms, somebody else is planning the strategy; you are planning the tactics. You've got short-term and medium-term troubles to deal with, and you've decided on the basic approach of spending a pittance on this book instead of $40,000 on an MBA degree. (Good choice!)

Set goals

The first thing to do is set a goal. As Jonathan's dad was known to observe, "Folks who don't know for sure where they are going usually end up not knowing where they are." Much has been written on goal-setting. It is, truly, the most important part of the planning process. Are you going to Orlando, or to Santa Fe? It makes a difference.

Goal setting is hard. Make it easy. Set goals that mean something to you. Don't worry if they don't sound like textbook examples, and don't worry if they might sound silly. "I want to be out of here by 5:30 p.m. at least four nights a week," is a *terrific* goal.

"I want to go six months without any employees quitting except those I secretly hoped would quit anyway," is a *terrific* goal. "I'd like to reduce the number of employee whining sessions that take place in my office to no more than two per week and the number of physician yelling sessions that take place in the hallway to no more than one per week," are *terrific* goals.

If those are your goals, you're staying late too often, you're running a department where turnover is a problem, and you're spending a lot of time dealing with anxious employees and angry physicians. Okay, call the current situation *here*. "Here" is our starting point. We want to get someplace called *there*, a place where the sun shines and the birds sing, where you go home on time, where employees don't quit all the time and where the level of stress has come down a peg or two.

We have to get from "here" to "there." Deciding how to do that is the first part of Axiom 8, the "Plan what you do" part. But the planning is worthless unless it is then turned into action. So we need a "Do what you plan" part. Without the plan *and* the action, it is all too easy to spend our days like Ed the Beagle, running first down one trail and then another until we stagger home at the end of the day, footsore, tired and hungry. Unlike Ed the Beagle, managers do not have the luxury of being carefree pups who can spend the day following interesting trails. Bosses actually expect our hunting to produce a catch.

What does success look like ...

The "there" we're heading for is the answer to the question, "What does success look like?" In medicine, as in any other business, success is a moving target, so that question must be asked and answered repeatedly, continually.

Let's now examine that question from several different vantage points. The perspectives we seek are: organizational, departmental and individual.

What does success look like for your organization?

Have you ever heard, "Our organization changes too fast for us to plan?" Or, "We are too busy doing the work to take the time to plan?" Those statements miss the point. They refer to techniques for developing a plan, not to the vision of success. Every organization has a definition of success, whether or not it grows out of applying a disciplined planning technique. That definition of success determines what to do and when to do it.

In this chapter we are less interested in the techniques and processes of planning, which are relatively easy, than we are interested in the definition of success, which is the hard part of planning. We are interested in answering the question, "What does success look like?" Remember Dr. Godley's definition? It didn't grow out of a disciplined planning process, but nonetheless, employees could understand it, sink their teeth into it and measure activities and results against it.

Whether stated or unstated, whether the result of a disciplined process or a tantrum, every organization defines what success looks like. What does success look like for your organization, as defined by those who control the power? Their definitions, not yours, drive the organization. They don't tell you? Sure they do. Some bosses tell it clearly in detail as a formal, written plan. Some tell it verbally and succinctly: "Get more money and keep more of the money we get!" Some hint at it: "We could really be a big operation in three years."

Direct communication from superiors is the best method of spreading the word, but if you've got your antennae out, you'll pick up even the faint signals that come from hints and suggestions, or even from rumor, gossip and innuendo. What's important is hearing the definition of success, verifying it with the boss, and then organizing people, resources and processes to achieve it.

By the way, whether your organization publishes a plan, or you absorb the plan by osmosis, bosses expect managers to understand and propagate the plan. And in truth, that's not expecting too much.

To meet those expectations, think about how your bosses define success, and put it in a brief written statement. No more than a few sentences. Include formal ideas as well as the unwritten notions of success. If there are no formal statements, use the following clues:

- What causes bosses to "go to pieces?" Avoiding the "go to pieces" issues is one type of success.

- Do the bosses make statements like this: "If we could just solve (blank), then we could really (blank)"? Removing those barriers and opening those doors is another form of success.

- When the bosses put their feet up and chat informally, what vision do they describe? "If we could get one contract with a manufacturer, we could use it to get into industrial medicine in a big way." These daydreams define success.

Think of these bits of information about future success as the pieces of a picture puzzle. You have the pieces, but you don't have the box they came in, so you don't know what the finished picture is supposed to look like. The challenge is to put the pieces together.

Now, here's the surprise. Everybody assumes that the rules of this game require you to use intuition and imagination to figure out what the picture is supposed to look like. You can do it that way if you want, but an easier way is to *ask the boss* what the darn thing is supposed to look like. Remember Axiom 7: Ask for help. Say to the boss, for example, "It seems to me we've been focusing more on industrial medicine lately. Is that true? Is that something that's going to be a big item for us?"

In five minutes of direct questioning you may learn more than you would in five weeks of nosing around.

At any rate, keep your eyes open. Pictures change. Sometimes, the same pieces have to be made into a totally different picture. Anyone who, for example, has had to comply with new regulations on short notice with no new budget can understand that challenge. Bosses have the right to expect as a minimum that managers will listen, think, see the obvious pieces of the puzzle, find the missing pieces and begin putting it all together.

The clues about future success may be few, obscure and even contradictory. So be it. Some bosses really make managers search. Still, the picture will begin to take shape after reflection. The next step is to verify that the boss wants the pieces to make a particular picture. One manager did it this way in a meeting. "I need to make sure that I'm working in the right directions. My understanding is that we want to accomplish X, Y and Z." The boss replied sarcastically, "No, I don't know where you got those ideas. We want to do F, G and H. You need to pay attention." Ah! One simple question produced exactly the information needed.

This particular manager was smarter than a beagle. When Jonathan spoke harshly to Ed about his hunting ability, Ed sulked into the dog house. If this manager had sulked when the boss spoke harshly, he would have lost opportunities. When you come to work, dress for success — wear the thickest skin you've got.

Even with a written plan, or perhaps especially with a written plan, managers must reflect on what success looks like for their organizations. They must then verify that picture of success and re-verify it regularly. They have to take the pieces available to them and put them together. Defining and verifying the picture keeps managers smarter than beagles. Otherwise, they hunt a lot of trails but never catch what the boss wants.

What does success look like for your part of the operation?

To use a previous example, if the task is to get the physician, the patient and the medical record in the room at the same time, what does your area contribute to it? What steps must your employees take? When must they take them? What rules, standards and laws must they follow? How do employees know when to adjust the process? How do you know when it is not working? These aren't all of the questions. Any manager can and should think of more.

Ask and answer these questions about your operation today. The answers define success (such as it is) for now. That helps define the "here." Then, ask and answer, "What does success look like in six months, 12 months and 24 months?" and ask the related questions in the paragraph above. These answers help define the "there" toward which you must go.

It is important to see your part of the operation in the proper perspective. Many people use the "choo choo" analogy to portray how the parts of an organization fit together and work together. They describe organizations as trains. The individual freight cars, passenger cars, baggage cars and mail cars are the departments of the organization. Each one has a separate function, but they're all tightly connected, all pulled along by the engine at the front, all traveling at the same speed and moving as a whole down the track. The engineer sets the course and speed. The whole train follows, busily clicking and merrily clacking. And, just as it was in *The Little Engine that Could*, no mountain is too steep for this brave train to climb, because the leader's determination inspires everyone into believing, "I think I can, I think I can."

Ha! It is more accurate to picture your organization as a vast fleet of ships, steaming out to sea and preparing to do battle with the enemy. Except in your case "steaming" is not quite the right word. Let's say "sort of" steaming, more or less out to sea, hoping to heaven that the enemy doesn't find us before we find them, because we're, um, not what you'd call "battle ready" just yet. But we can be ready tomorrow, or the next day for sure. At least we think we can, we think we can.

With their common mission being to engage the enemy, every ship in the fleet is headed in pretty much the same direction. But unlike train cars, the ships are spread out, and not all headed in exactly the same direction at any moment. And while most of the ships are pounding the waves and making progress toward some ultimate goal, some are going faster than others. And some ships are not doing well: one has engine problems, one has a busted rudder, one is dead in the water, one is listing and one is headed back to port for fear of sinking.

Goodness, and this is all before the enemy has even been sighted!

How does this naval analogy relate to the topic of this chapter? It has to do with an earlier point: probably someone other than you is planning the *strategies* for the organization. That person is the admiral or the fleet commander in this analogy; you and other front-line managers are the captains of ships. You are planning *tactics* more than strategies. You have to know how to do your part, within the framework of the bigger picture.

In a big fleet, each ship is a functional unit with a specific responsibility. Some tasks can be shared, such as transporting supplies and personnel, but other tasks are discrete and simply cannot be shared: you can't ask the mine sweepers to do the aircraft carriers' job. In your organization, departments (and sometimes even individual people) are the functional units, with discrete responsibilities. You can't expect the mail room supervisor to do the bookkeeper's job, no matter how good that mail room supervisor is.

You are the captain of your ship. You and your department have certain responsibilities nobody else shares. And just as the ships in an armada are not strongly interconnected, neither are the departments in your organization. They share an overall mission, but they run somewhat independently. You have to move with the fleet, but you have to keep your own ship afloat.

Of course there's some admiral in some stateroom on some command ship in the middle of the flotilla, three miles away, giving you orders. That's completely proper. But the admiral can't see what is actually happening where *you* are. *You've* got eight foot seas and open hatches. *You've* got balky generators and faulty bilge pumps. *You've* got hungry sailors and a drunken cook.

You see the point. "Success" from the admiral's perspective is different from success as a ship's captain sees it. Success for an admiral may mean routing the enemy and losing "only" five ships.

For a captain, losing only one ship could be a total disaster — if it is that captain's ship.

Similarly, success is one thing for a hospital's executive board; it's one thing for a medical staff president; it's one thing for a private group's owner/physicians — and it is another for us as their managers. Their view may encompass your view, but it won't coincide precisely. Their view should be more strategic, more long-term, than yours as a manager. You need to understand their view of success and you need to support their mission — while keeping your department floating, achieving tactical successes and keeping your aft out of the water.

What does success look like for your people?

Don't make your employees work the way Ed the Beagle had to hunt — without directions from his boss. Managers who find themselves saying an employee "has been here long enough to figure out what to do" make the same mistake Jonathan made. He thought Ed could figure it out for himself. As Jonathan's father said, "If a person won't teach a dog to hunt rabbits, there's no complaint when the dog can't find them."

One manager we know meets with her employees each week and defines what success looks like for the next week. Again, she specifies goals that make sense to the group, and she uses simple language. "No misfiled X-rays this week" is a terrific goal. She asks the staff what they need from her to achieve success and what barriers might be in the way. She asks them to verbalize how they will approach the tasks. With a clear picture, the employees can put the puzzle together.

This approach to managing changed her use of time and her conversations with employees. Once the employees knew what to do, she could spend more time obtaining resources, removing barriers and coaching individual employees. Previously, she had spent time asking why things were not done, engaging in frustrating conversations and fussing at employees. A pretty good change, don't you think?

Her boss was not as clear. In fact, her boss was anything but clear and polite in conversations. But managers manage many things. (Sometimes we simply manage to get through the day.) This manager saw part of her management role as calming the uproar from her boss, and translating his uncertainty into consistency and direction, through considerate discussion with her employees. When the boss changed directions, she translated the changes for minimum disruptions. Wow! She sat on her thoughts about how the boss "ought" to do things, believing an obligation to do so came with the territory. And she knew that if the day ever came when she was no longer willing to stay in that territory, she would move on to another.

When employees know what success looks like, they are more likely to achieve it. When they have to guess, they make their best guess. But, because it is a guess, their actions lack confidence. They spend a lot of time figuring out what to say if they are questioned. They resent not receiving instructions. What does success look like for employees? Answering that question can change the way they spend their time and energy.

In a crisis, one clinic manager said, "Here's what we need to do today." Then he gave specific instructions, and said, "Don't worry about anything else. If we accomplish just this, we will have had a successful day and we all can hold our heads high. No matter what else happens, remember, all we have to do today is what we discussed. We will start the rest tomorrow." Instead of being overwhelmed by the crisis, defining and achieving an increment of success enabled the employees to take charge of the crisis. Using incremental definitions of success moved them successfully from "here" to "there." And as a side benefit, it was a simple demonstration of one of the fundamentals of planning.

It does not take much imagination to know what happens when managers teach employees that kind of basic technique. It is like using a really good tool for, say, opening all those shipping cartons and plastic bags we get at work. Let people see you using it, then leave it lying around. Soon everyone uses it. Not only that, they look for other tools for other tasks. One way to approach management is to find good tools, demonstrate their use and leave them lying around. If the tools are good, most people have the sense to use them.

So: tell employees what success looks like from your perspective and ask them what it looks like to them.

Then what?

After all this questioning and answering — which we said earlier was the hard part — what do you do? You figure out the sequence and the priorities, write everything down and get to work. For many people this part of the planning process is much easier than setting goals. Once you get this far along in the process, things become more concrete. The targets stop moving. Everyday skills can be applied.

Everyday skills? Like what?

Like the "sequencing and prioritizing" skills you developed from years of grocery shopping, meal-planning and cooking, for example.

Ever have a card party at your house, or plan a baby shower, or organize a softball league? Have you ever planned a simple, tasteful breakfast — for 250 wedding guests?

These are things that ordinary people do successfully in their personal lives. Some of these things call for pretty sophisticated planning, and require well-honed abilities to do what professionals call "sequencing and prioritizing."

Creating a plan of action, whether it is for business or pleasure, means listing all the required steps, being sure the sequence is correct, and setting priorities. It is not a hard thing to conceptualize and in fact it is often not a hard thing to do. If you take the time to list all the steps, the sequence is often self-evident.

Take the time to list all the steps.

A good drill for your employees is to get them together as a group and make a list of what tasks must be tackled to have a card party at home. Just start writing as people call out items for the list. The start of the list will probably look something like this:

- ✓ buy chips (potato and betting)
- ✓ beer, cards
- ✓ get a pooch sitter
- ✓ clean up the living room
- ✓ get the stereo fixed
- ✓ invite everybody (who? when?)
- ✓ warn the neighbors & police this time
- ✓ enough chairs? tablecloth?
- ✓ make snacks, or send out for pizza?

Eventually the list may include several dozen items. Just like the plans you make at work, this list will end up mentioning only three basic categories: people, things and time. After all, what else is there?

Prioritize the steps.

When everyone is satisfied with the list, make a copy for each person, and ask them individually to number the tasks according to what must be done first, second, last. Compare lists and discuss variations. You'll find some defensible matters of preference expressed — some people will want to make the bean dip three days ahead of time and some will prefer doing it right before the guests arrive — but it is unusual to find answers that truly don't make sense. For instance, you won't find anyone listing "invite the guests" as one of the *last* steps.

Rate the steps according to importance.

Ask everyone to rate the items on their list as to their importance to the success of the party, on a scale of A, B, C, D, E. This is where the fun begins. Some people say, "Everything is important!" Others say things like, "You need people and you need cards. Everything else is secondary. Well, you do need beer." What people say will depend partly on their own mental picture of a successful card party, and partly (as we discussed in Axiom 5) on whether they are "process-oriented" or "results-oriented."

Cut your list in half.

Now, finally, change the rules. Tell them, "We can't do all the things on this list. Our 'things' budget was just cut 50 percent. We have to re-do this list, knocking out 50 percent of it. I don't mean 50 percent of the money the party would cost, I just mean cross out half the items on this list, and still come up with a way to have a card party. We have to work as a group to get this done."

In other words, we want to force people into thinking really hard about what is important. The people who said "Everything is important" will groan. The minimalists will say, "Easy. Keep the people, the cards and the beer." *Between them,* they'll probably come up with a pretty darned good list. And that is precisely the point. Effective planning requires getting the sequence right (easy) and the priorities right (hard). The planning process works best when you are careful to involve people with different outlooks.

Summary

When you stare long enough at a list of tasks, a plan will eventually form, like a photograph materializing in a developing tray. Many managers are afraid to spend the quiet time required to make this happen. They are afraid to be still, to stare, to mull and to ponder. They'd be embarrassed if someone ever caught them pondering.

Don't you be like that.

Spend the time it takes to plan! Every minute spent planning will save a minimum of 312.5 minutes later on, according to our highly accurate scientific survey. Do your own highly accurate survey and compare results.

Why bother planning? It's how to get things done. Getting things done is what managers are paid to do. And there is another reason: planning helps to focus and direct everyone's energies.

Every organization, and everybody in it, is on a journey every day, from some here to some there. You can dictate where you're going, or you can be carried along anonymously by the dull momentum of events. It's much more fun to take an active role, to make your journey an adventure of daily progress toward a definite goal. Arriving at a goal is great, but getting there is half the fun.

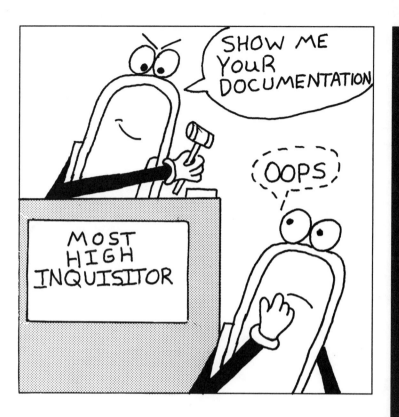

AXIOM 9

Get it in writing

C heck out the tabloids at the supermarket: "A Martian is the father of my children." "Three-headed calf delivers message from God." "Paranoid clerk discovered in musty mail room." "I cloned my wife from my mother's fingernail clippings."

In this chapter we will discuss business documentation. We'll take a look at some of the why's and what's and how's of documentation, as well as some of the why not's and what not's and how not's. We have begun at a perfectly logical place, at the supermarket, where each week we see a new array of strange and wonderful headlines. They lure us and compel us to spend an extra buck and "read all about it." Why begin there? To illustrate a few quick points about how to write and what to write.

First, though, think for a moment about the quantity and variety of things that are documented in a medical organization — things such as patient records, financial data, agendas and minutes of meetings, personnel and payroll files, and safety, training and compliance manuals, just to name a few. And then reflect on how much trouble can be caused by improper documentation — trouble such as malpractice and discrimination lawsuits, Medicare "fraud and abuse" investigations and IRS audits, just to name a few. You can see that "documentation" is an immensely broad and important topic.

Back to the tabloids. Have you figured out there's a ringer in the headlines above? It's the one that says, "Paranoid clerk discovered in musty mail room." That didn't come from a supermarket tabloid, it came from a note one of your authors saw in a personnel file. Really.

Okay, okay, the actual handwritten note didn't say, "Paranoid clerk discovered in musty mail room." It said simply, "Jim is paranoid." But if you were an EEOC investigator looking for evidence of discrimination, that little note would be every bit as compelling as a tabloid headline. You would want to read all about it. You'd want to investigate *very* thoroughly, to learn how a psychological condition as complex as paranoia could have been diagnosed with such certainty by the mail room supervisor who wrote the note and who was presumably not a trained psychiatrist. You'd want to know if the supervisor, believing Jim to be paranoid, acted differently toward him, perhaps downgrading his performance evaluations or overlooking him for promotions. You'd want to know if the supervisor ever said "Jim" and "paranoia" in the same breath to another employee.

And so on and so on. In other words, you'd want to make as much trouble as possible.

What a difference a phrase makes. If the supervisor's note had read "Jim *says he's* 'paranoid'" instead of "Jim *is* paranoid," the entire picture changes. Instead of being an inflammatory accusation, "Jim says he's 'paranoid'" is simply a quotation. Any baggage that comes with the statement is Jim's, not the supervisor's. At *worst* such a note might lead to a standoff in which Jim denies having made the remark and the supervisor simply stands by the accuracy of the written record.

"House dust cures cancer!" the tabloid screams. Please. Aren't there any rules for writing stuff like that? *Sure* there are. The publishers (and their lawyers) probably know the rules by heart. We don't, but let's take a guess. Tabloid Rule Number One surely must be: mislead the reader. The trickier the headline the better. The harder it is for the reader to separate fact from fiction, the better.

Anything wrong with that? Naaa. Everybody knows (or ought to know) that supermarket tabloids are misleading. That's a big part of the fun. It's perverse, certainly. It's like going to horror movies to be scared stiff and calling *that* fun. It's that same perversity that causes us to read outrageous tabloid fiction and pretend it might be true.

But on the other hand, we become indignant at the merest suspicion that a "real" newspaper or a respected news magazine might be careless with the truth. And the notion that they might *intentionally* mislead us is simply unthinkable. That would violate a sacred trust.

Okay, let's review, to be sure we've got this right: misleading the reader is allowed and even encouraged in one type of writing, but misleading the reader is outrageous and unthinkable in another type of writing. Right? Yes, that's right. Those are the rules.

Guidelines for documentation

So, what are the rules for the kind of documentation managers do? An excellent question! And here's the answer: *it depends.* Does it ever depend!

On the topic of documentation it is easy to become overwhelmed, and easy to be "confused with the facts." As managers, what we *don't* need is an enormous list that attempts to define the precise documentation requirements of our specific business. Instead, we are much better served by knowing general principles that can be applied to specific situations. We need "guiding lights," meaning we need reliable advice to keep our thoughts on track when we face thorny questions about documentation. Here are some guiding lights:

- If it's not written down it didn't happen.

- Writing it down doesn't mean it happened.

- Writing it down doesn't make it happen.

- Writing it down can sink you.

- Not writing it down can sink you.

- Write it down to clear it up.

- Block that metaphor!

- Hold that bus!

Those items, you may have guessed, are subtopics in this chapter. After explaining each of those, we'll turn our attention to some why's and how's.

A quick note before we begin. When we talk about "writing," we mean every type and method of documentation there ever was, is, or will be: from stone tablets to floptical disks, from papyrus to voice mail, from napkin doodles to virtual reality. It's all the same for the purposes of this chapter: it's all "written down."

If it's not written down it didn't happen

This expression is often used as an explanation of why someone is unwilling to take another person's word for something. For example, in a malpractice case, the physician says, "I vividly remember giving the order for the antidote."

"Did you write the orders? Are the orders in the chart?" asks the prosecuting attorney, handing the physician "Exhibit B."

The physician barely looks. He has seen it before. "Apparently not. But I do remember it clearly," says the physician.

"Doctor, do you know the meaning of the phrase, 'If it's not written down it didn't happen'?" asks the attorney.

Oops! The physician is about to get an expensive lesson, one that follows this logic: Things that are not well-documented are hard to prove; things that are hard to prove are easy to contradict; if what you say can be easily contradicted, you're probably lying through your teeth.

Wait! Is that fair? No, that's life. Important statements and decisions and events need to be documented. Period. A quick note in the chart would have prevented this "oops."

Here's another example. Linda was late 13 times in one month. She responded to warnings by saying, "I will be on time." More tardiness. A final warning. Termination. But no one wrote any of this down. When Linda complained to a government agency, she said, "No one told me being late could cost me my job."

"Yes, I did. We talked three times," her supervisor says at the hearing.

"When?" asks the agency representative.

"I don't remember the exact dates."

"Show me your documentation," the representative requests, adding, "Because around here we believe, 'If it's not written down it didn't happen.'"

Oops! Documenting each incident when it happened, with the employee receiving a copy, would have prevented this "oops!"

Good documentation not only helps protect you against external threats such as lawsuits and investigations, but it also helps protect you from internal problems. For example, imagine this:

The key people met and discussed purchasing video training programs, complete with expensive video cassette players. No one disagreed with the necessity of the training or the purchase. You place the order. Eight weeks later the business manager sees the invoice and goes through the roof. You say, "But you agreed to this in the meeting." The business manager, whose concerns over cash flow have obviously altered his memory, says, "I agreed to the concept. I certainly did not agree to spend the money. We can't spend money like that in a fiscal quarter like this one." *Oops.*

A memorandum to those who attended the meeting could have prevented this oops. Something like, "This memorandum summarizes the conclusions we reached in the meeting of mm/dd/yy concerning the video training." The memo would list the conclusions, one, two, three, four, etc., in simple sentences. One of the conclusions is the agreement to spend the money. The closing says, "Let me know if you have a different understanding of any of the conclusions. I will place the order in three days unless there is reason to re-think our decision."

Good documentation means never having to say "Oops!" Doing the right thing isn't enough: you have to do the right thing, *and be able to prove you did it.*

Before we leave "If it's not written down it didn't happen," let's mention that the meaning of this expression changes significantly, depending on whether it is used to support something someone *claims,* as opposed to supporting something someone *denies.* Above, we used the phrase to show how written records can support your word or your memory, and can help prove that what you claim is true. But the opposite can also apply: if you deny something, and if there is no written record to contradict you, your denial is supported by the lack of documentation. You get to say, "Nyaaa nyaaa, if it isn't written down it didn't happen."

Sometimes people intentionally avoid making written statements *because* an authentic written record is permanent and irrefutable. Sometimes people shun documentation because writing tends to clarify issues, and with clarity comes accountability. Sometimes people refuse to leave a "paper trail" so they can reinvent history as it suits them at any point in time. For example, Dr. Godley wants nothing in writing. When he tells the history and war stories of his clinic, he doesn't want the drama to be inhibited by the facts.

That sounds quaint, but it can also be dangerous. If we were talking about politics, this topic would be called "deniability." The word and the concept seem sinister, and they certainly can be. In plain English, "deniability" can mean lying, and lying is normally to be avoided.

True. And yet, consider the following:

As a manager, sometimes you learn things you'd be better off not knowing— things you don't want others to discover you're aware of. When that happens, you are not required to put a noose around your own neck. Do yourself a favor and don't make records of the details.

This is an area that can present agonizing questions of ethics and judgment, but here's an example that doesn't go to extremes. Let's say you're walking past the smokers' lounge, and you hear someone saying, "Did you see Lottie's new sweater? She probably bought it with the money she stole from petty cash." Laughter erupts.

Keep walking while you think this through. Yes, the money was missing — enough to buy a sweater — and Lottie did have access to it. And Lottie *can* be secretive, perhaps even suspicious.

On the other hand, Lottie is not popular with the younger workers and she's frequently the target of potshots just like this. And for all you know, this might just be a joke: Lottie might have been right there *in the lounge,* hearing the same thing you heard; Lottie's best friend may have said it to her face — something so obviously and outrageously impossible that everyone would find it funny. Maybe that's all this was ... Still, what was said contained a serious accusation.

Now the kicker: Overlying this whole thing is the important fact that Lottie is due for retirement next month.

So, are you going to do anything? Maybe, maybe not. You have to decide for yourself.

Would we (the authors) do anything? Naaa. We'd lock up the cash, keep a sharp watch on Lottie and just ride this problem out. Are we going to write down *anything, anywhere,* about this? Naaa. *No good can come from it,* and we might be setting a trap for ourselves by documenting our unfounded (and unacted-upon) suspicions.

Writing it down doesn't mean it happened

Speaking of lying, as we were earlier, you don't think anyone would ever *make up* something, do you, and then create documentation to try to prove it happened when actually it didn't? And you don't think anyone would ever try to pass off reconstructed documents as originals, do you?

Sure they would. Happens all the time. That's why the really hard-nosed, suspicious, cynical, cold-hearted disbelievers of this world — including the authors of this book — live by the corollary, "Writing it down doesn't mean it happened." Just because someone is able to show a written record doesn't mean the record is authentic. The record *itself* has to be proven. Sheesh, what next? The proof has to be verified? The verification has to be authenticated? No, not really. In the practical world there's an end to all this. Most of the time, documentation is taken at face value; otherwise, nobody would ever get anything done. But the point of this guideline is this: Whenever there's a lot at stake, you can bet someone will question the accuracy or authenticity of the record. So the record had better be solid.

"Did you write the orders? Are the orders in the chart?" asks the prosecuting attorney, handing the physician "Exhibit B."

The physician barely looks. He has seen it before. "Yes. Right there," says the physician.

"And *when* did you make this chart notation, Doctor? At the time of the incident, or later, as in *much* later, as in after this lawsuit was filed?"

Objection! The prosecutor is being a hard-nosed, suspicious, cynical, cold-hearted disbeliever. Overruled. That's life.

Creating an entirely phony record is probably rare; writing things down from memory, long after the actual events, is much more common and is what we will focus on here. The need for reconstruction comes from failing to document properly at the time.

Here's a story almost identical to the "Late Linda" story we saw earlier in this chapter, except this time there's documentation available to substantiate the supervisor's version of events. The characters in this story are Ms. Short, who was a supervisor; Tom, an undependable employee; and Tim, Tom's friend and co-worker.

Ms. Short was aptly named. No, she stood five feet ten, so it wasn't her height that made her name the source of an occasional snicker; it was the fact that she was "short" and abrupt in conversations with employees. She was also short-tempered and short-sighted.

Ms. Short fired Tom for being late once too often. He filed a complaint, saying, she "… treated me unfairly, did not like me, fired me for no reason, did not fire other employees who did the same thing, and was out to get me from the very beginning."

The government agency politely asked Ms. Short to be so kind as to provide copies of all documentation of conversations with the employee leading up to the firing. And would she be so kind as to provide copies of all documentation of disciplinary actions against other employees who were disciplined in similar circumstances? And would she also provide a race/gender/age/religion analysis of current employees, terminated employees and applicants for employment for the last three years? All within two weeks, if you don't mind.

She didn't have any of the documentation requested. *Oops.* So she decided to create it. That gets a "5" on the "oops" meter.

Ms. Short called her employees together and asked them to help her reconstruct the events leading to Tom's dismissal so she could write the report. She did not mislead anyone, then or later. She didn't claim the record was contemporaneous and she never tried to pretend it was anything other than a reconstruction.

As it turns out she might as well have saved her time. She found out at the hearing that Tim called Tom and said, "Ms. Short asked all the employees to talk against you." Tim himself quit the day before the hearing, and repeated his statement at the hearing, saying he felt forced to quit before Ms. Short "got me the way she got Tom."

Ms. Short's reconstruction of the events was accurate; her documentation was impeccable; what she wrote down actually happened. But the hearing officer was a strong believer in the phrase, "Writing it down doesn't mean it happened." Tim's statement supported Tom's contentions. Plus, Ms. Short openly stated she created the documentation after the fact. As far as the agency was concerned, what she had written was irrelevant. It was taken from memory, after the passage of time. Written or not, it was still from memory. Writing it down did not make it a better record than Tom and Tim's memory. In the agency's eyes the record had been effectively challenged and was now tarnished.

This story did not have a happy ending for Ms. Short, whose tenure with the organization also turned out to be short. And the organization itself suffered, being made to reinstate lazy Tom and malcontented Tim. With back pay, of course.

The time to record things is *as soon after they occur as you can,* while they are fresh in your mind. Even contemporaneous documentation is open to challenge, but at least it cannot be dismissed as faulty memory.

Reconstructing events and writing documentation after the fact is difficult, ineffective, dangerous, and possibly illegal, depending on the issue. In particular, don't ever go back and add anything to a medical record without clearly annotating who, when and why the addition was made. And if something in a medical record must be changed (as opposed to added to), don't erase or white out or cover up the original information. Make a single line through it, make the correction, and date, initial and explain the reason for the alteration. Doing these things improperly can lose lawsuits and licenses and can provide extended time away from the clinic in less-than-luxurious surroundings.

In the story above, the outcome might easily have been the same even without Tim's phone call. Experienced agency staff are trained to mistrust re-created stories. And they can "sniff out" phony documentation, so don't even think about trying that.

Post-event documentation can not overcome memory gaps and the tendency to rewrite history. The passage of time increases the discrepancies among the accounts of the event. Like it or not, agencies tend to be advocates of the people who come to them. Like it or not, employers have the burden of disproving fired employee's allegations. Documenting appropriately as events unfold is a sure cure for the problem of reconstructing events.

Even the best observers see the same events differently; even people with excellent memories revise and edit after the fact. Civil war history provides an excellent example of both tendencies. Pickett's charge at Gettysburg resulted in conflicting accounts by Generals Lee, Longstreet, Pickett and Hood. Each outlined different reasons for the charge, and their accounts vary considerably as to the preliminary estimates each made of the artillery cover needed in advance of the charge, and as to when the artillery actually appeared, if at all. Jeb Stuart and the cavalry were not in the right place at the right time, with disastrous results for the South. Stuart faced serious accusations after the battle. John Mosby wrote a book attempting to exonerate Stuart 30 years after the event. Surprise! It differs from almost every report written at the time.

This military analogy is apt. Documentation provides the ammunition for battles such as malpractice suits, reimbursement squabbles, unemployment compensation claims, disciplinary actions, and investigations of complaints of discrimination and harassment, to name a few. Write it as it happens. You don't have time not to write it down. Writing it down after the fact does not mean it happened.

Writing it down doesn't make it happen

In the movie *Evil Roy Slade*, a spoof of the old west, the outlaw Evil Roy Slade falls in love with the local schoolmarm. He instructs his accountant, "Give me $50,000 to start a new life with Betsy, and divide the rest among the boys." The accountant shows him the ledger and says, "But, boss, we don't have $50,000. In fact we don't have *any* money."

With a threatening sneer, Evil Roy says, "You write a five in that book and a bunch of zeroes until it says 'fifty thousand dollars.'" The accountant complies. Evil Roy then says, "*Now* give it to me."

Of course writing it down did not make it happen. Evil Roy had to rob a stage coach to get his nest egg. Too often, managers make the same mistake: They think that because they wrote the instructions, something happened. When writing it down does not make it happen, like Evil Roy, they have to take drastic action to recover.

Confirm verbal messages in writing, simply to assure the message was received. But just because people receive messages doesn't mean they're going to do anything else. Follow-up is essential. Writing it down does not make it happen.

It is tempting to think that our clear and brilliantly written memos cause the results we want, but chances are the memos are just more fodder for the system. What system? The system that loses, ignores and eats memos. Every office has one. You know it works well when people say, "I didn't know that," "I didn't see a memo on that," or "I wasn't notified." The system is operated by persons such as the "Experienced Executive Secretary" who put copies of an important memo in the personnel files of nine individuals but never delivered the memo to any one of them personally. We have all heard of a mail clerk who got tired of delivering mail and tossed it in the trash. These incidents show the system functioning at its best.

Even when the message gets through and a confirmation comes back and good things begin to happen, follow up to make sure your expectations are being met. Writing it down does not make it happen: prodding and inspecting and complaining and begging and threatening—you know, all the regular management techniques—those things make it happen.

Dr. Godley's clinic administrator developed a plan for converting unused lobby space into office space. Financial reality required putting up the walls during one fiscal year and then using whatever furniture could be scrounged up until the next fiscal year, when a bunch of modular cubicles and new furniture could be bought.

The plan was approved and distributed, the walls went up and the staff moved in. It was ugly but functional and would do for the three months remaining in the current fiscal year.

Three months into the new fiscal year it was still ugly. But "ugly" was not the problem. Nobody remembered to order the cubicles and furniture, which were needed to double up on the number of people who could work in the area. The additional people currently occupied space needed for the new computer. The whole reason for converting the lobby space was to make room for the computer, which was now on a truck, on its way to the clinic. *Oops.*

Writing it down did not make it happen. Without follow up, the project had been stalled.

Writing it down can sink you

An eager manager took it upon herself to become the clinic's authority on implementing "universal precautions." No one else wanted the duty, and Dr. Godley approved of her interest. As the deadline for implementation approached, she distributed manuals defining procedures and assigning responsibilities. One by one, the other department managers walked into her office and took her head off.

To each one she protested, "But it has to be done and nobody else wanted to do it, and my manual is sound." Each one replied, "That's right, but you should have consulted me before distributing it. I have some thoughts about it, too." She finally got the point: memos and other written documents should rarely tell key people anything new; they should confirm the consensus that has already been reached.

Written communication is not the best way to initiate dialogue or inform others, unless you are the Big Boss. The Big Boss is not always right, but is always the Big Boss. Those who are not the Big Boss must talk to key people to build consensus. Building consensus involves discussions, recommendations, revisions and all the other time-consuming give-and-take. Only after that is done should a written document confirm what everyone already knows.

Even after building consensus, the *way* you write can sink you. If your written communication appears to violate the pecking order, infringe on another's territory, present you as an "insider" or otherwise indicate a view that does not square with reality, it can sink you.

Writers publicly commit to the impressions their documents create, for good or ill. You may have heard the expression, "He can't give you a gold brick without making you mad." Some people write the same way. Most writers stop at one, and usually three, re-writes short of a finished version. Most writers distribute their work too soon. Some overdo it. They document in the same way one patient took digitalis for her heart condition: one tablet made her feel so good that she took two and nearly killed herself. Others document the way a lot of people take allergy shots: the first one doesn't seem to do any good, so they quit. Still others document the way over-the-counter medicine junkies take remedies: they take one of everything, creating a combination that has disastrous effects.

Moral: too much or too little are equally ineffective, and the wrong thing or wrong combination can be disastrous.

Here's an example of someone getting sunk by writing it down:

Ms. Short was annoyed with the physicians for several reasons, including not showing up on time, which threw the lunch schedule off. One day her frustration spilled over and she wrote a heated memo directly to the medical director, who was two levels above her in the organization. She pointed out that her employees were always on time, but the physicians were *never* on time.

Any ideas about the reaction of the medical director? He granted her a short meeting, and he had two short words for her: "Prove it." She couldn't. She had no documentation. He reminded her that if it's not written down it didn't happen, and he sent her on her way.

Rule: Don't ever send a memo you write when your fuse is short and burning. If your position is valid, it can be stated calmly and appropriately later.

Here's yet another way you can sink yourself by writing it down: put something in writing you are reluctant to say face-to-face. Bad news, expressions of disagreement or other communications of an unpleasant nature are generally more palatable when delivered face-to-face. As adults, not to mention as managers, we must simply accept and uphold this difficult standard of behavior. Few statements express more contempt than to say, "Les Spine didn't have the nerve to tell me to my face; he put it in a memo."

Anger, especially, should be delivered face-to-face. A memo expressing anger is almost always a mistake. In the cold light of review, an exchange of hostile memos stirs up images of spoiled children pointing fingers.

Some people swear by the therapeutic value of writing a hostile note or letter and then throwing it in the trash. Or sleeping on it, revising it carefully and *then* throwing it in the trash. As firm believers in "Writing it down can sink you," the authors advise against this practice. Go to the gym and work out your aggression. If you must write something you intend never to send, be sure it never *ever* sees the light of day.

Worth repeating: don't write to inform other managers — it strains the relationships. Write to document the consensus that already exists. Face-to-face communication can take a lot of energy and can be aggravating, but managers cannot avoid those costs. The task is unavoidable. Face-to-face communication is unavoidable. You can do it now, or you can do it later, but you have to do it. If you write it down when you ought to communicate in person, writing it down can sink you.

Not writing it down can sink you

Didn't we just say the opposite of this? Yes. That's one reason why documentation is so hard: You can do the right thing for the wrong reason, or vice versa, and you're in trouble. Proper documentation takes careful thought and good judgment.

Much of the concept "Not writing it down can sink you" overlaps what was covered earlier, in the discussion about "If it's not written down it didn't happen." In that earlier section, clearly, people who didn't write things down had their word questioned, *and they were sunk.* In this section we want to show your good intentions are no more valuable than your word. Even when people truly believe what you say, if you can't produce the documentation they often cannot act in your behalf.

Back to Ms. Short, who by now must look to you like someone who never learns from past mistakes — or at the least suffered from a short memory. In this episode she sank herself by not keeping good notes or records.

Remember her short meeting with the medical director? She didn't give up after that. She decided to "accentuate the positive" instead of focusing on the negative. She told her boss she could demonstrate how the clinic could see 12 more patients a day with no increase in overhead.

That would be pure profit, she figured. And she also figured that in order to get this profit, some of the physicians would have to change unproductive work habits — the very habits that were causing them to run late. Finally, Ms. Short recognized that she had burned her bridges with the medical director, so she would have to enlist the support of her own boss, who would in turn have to enlist the support of the medical director. Still, the plan looked workable, and very much worth the effort.

All this was actually very good thinking on her part. Ms. Short was not a slow learner. She understood timing, packaging, planning ... Her tragic flaw was her lack of understanding and appreciation about proper documentation.

Because he had a strong notion she was right about increasing productivity, her boss was willing to go to bat for her — providing she could document her contention that, "If the physicians would stop doing procedures that medical assistants could do, the physicians would be much more likely to stay on schedule. And if they ran on time, we wouldn't have to send an average of 12 patients a day to the ER for care we could provide here."

He asked her to keep a log of each occurrence—who, what, when and where. Six weeks passed. Then one day her boss walked in, looking pleased. He said he'd just had a nice informal chat with the medical director and had suggested to him that there might be an opportunity "to streamline patient flow" and perhaps see more patients.

"This is it," her boss said. "Here's our chance. Where's your log?"
Oops!

She timidly confessed that she had quit documenting because, "Nothing was changing and I was too busy to write all that stuff down."

She was sunk. Period. Completely down the tubes, with *no chance* of recovery. She also undercut her boss's ability to help solve the problem. And she undercut his credibility and her own. He was never able to address the problem.

Write it down to clear it up

One obvious and useful meaning of this phrase is that if you write your instructions down, there will be less confusion about what you meant by them. Write them down to clear them up. Enough said.

But the meaning we're after is less obvious, and it applies to the *writer*, not the recipient. Here it is: writing helps clarify your own thoughts. When your thinking is a little fuzzy on an issue, write about it — to help clear up your thoughts.

Writing is hard. Writing demands discipline and clear thinking. Many of us are brain lazy; anything that imposes discipline and clear thinking is good for us. Writing does just that.

Jotting notes or dictating notes preserves important ideas for later use. But like seedlings, these ideas die without nurturing. Writing them out fully helps to develop them for your own benefit, even if no one else sees them. Writing forces completion of thought; it disciplines logic and it requires spelling out of assumptions. It also exposes what's missing. Writing develops insights.

A few hours each month spent in reviewing operations and writing descriptions of the organization — where it is now, where it should be in three months, the barriers to getting there and what you will do to remove the barriers — can be valuable. Even if you send it to no one, these musings have done their job. They've made you use your mind.

Block that metaphor!

Before we move on to the "hows" of writing, let's deal with fear. Many managers would rather do anything other than write. They believe writing is something normal people don't do, at least not in public. In their secret heart they believe writing is sorcery.

This is a chapter about documentation, not about the art of writing. But it is important for us to confront the widespread fear of writing, because our advice about documentation may produce nothing but frustration and feelings of inadequacy among managers who have a mental block against writing. People fear writing because as a subject it is full of hateful and confusing things, such as grammar, spelling, sentence structure, the difference between metaphor and simile, and so on.

If you suffer from a fear of writing, the good news is that nobody expects you to write a novel, for goodness' sake. You have to be able to write a readable memo, proposal, summary of a plan, or a clear and concise note in a personnel file. Even these are not a cakewalk, but they are within the grasp of most people. Like most other things we have discussed in this book, this isn't all that complicated.

More good news. You can overcome your dread of writing if you take just these two steps: 1) write anyway and 2) ask for help.

Like marathon runners who must run "through the pain," if you intend to write, you must simply write. Not study writing, not dictate, not anything else. Nothing else substitutes. You must put pen to paper (or fingertips to keyboard) and compose, edit, review, re-write — write. Now, you certainly don't have to show what you've written to anyone if you don't want to, but you *do* have to write.

Yes, it might hurt. Writing is hard for many people. That's why those who can do a passable job of it have a big advantage over those who can't.

The next step is, eventually, to ask for help. The traditional advice is to go to the community college and take a business writing class, or go to the library or bookstore and read up on the topic. Fine. But for practical purposes it is just as effective simply to ask a superior at work to review drafts of things you've written before you file or distribute them. Pick someone who knows what they're doing and whose own writing is clear and concise, and ask for help. Trust us: people are flattered when someone appreciates their writing. They'll be glad to advise you.

Memorize this rule: "Simplify, simplify." That's Thoreau's advice, and it sums up everything most of us ever need to know about business writing. Don't use a long word when a short one will do. Use short sentences that make solid statements. Don't get tricky, flowery, clever or funny. Block that metaphor! In other words, don't strive for vivid images in your business writing. Get the facts down on paper, and get on with your other important work.

Hold that bus!

You need a standard for documenting work in progress. Here it is. It's simple: Document so that if a manager is hit by a bus, anyone can go to the files and know the following items quickly:

- the projects and what is at stake in each project;
- the state of completion of each project;
- the issues to be resolved;
- what remains to be done; and
- who is accountable.

Many organizations don't know it, but they are one automobile accident or one serious illness away from total dysfunction. *Oops!*

A quick, important tip: proposals and memos should always be marked "DRAFT; FOR DISCUSSION ONLY" unless they truly are the truly final version. *Truly.* Marking them as "drafts" keeps you from having to defend them as legitimate policy if the memos fall into the wrong hands.

That completes the "guiding lights" section of this chapter. Now we will briefly discuss some of the "how's and what's" of documentation.

How to write what down

There's an old story told to law students about a man having a heart attack who scribbled three words on a scrap of paper, signed it and dropped dead. The note said, "All to wife," and it stood up in court as a valid will. (And as his last will, obviously.)

Whew. A very close call. There's a proper way to prepare a will, and that isn't it. There's a proper way of documenting everything. There's a proper way, an acceptable way, a passable way; and then there are close calls, nice tries and "oopses." As a manager you need to know, in detail, what the documentation requirements are for your area and who's responsible for meeting those requirements. A book like this can't begin to describe in detail what is needed at your organization. You will have to figure it out for yourself. Luckily there's help.

For those of you with money to spend, here's the short course: call your attorneys and get them to come snoop around and make recommendations about "how to write what down." *This is money well spent.*

For do-it-yourselfers, many people and organizations stand ready to give you advice, including the Internal Revenue Service, the American Medical Association, your local medical society, Medical Group Management Association, your boss, your malpractice carrier and your accountant. In addition, articles appear regularly in the trade periodicals on this topic. All you need to do is open your eyes, and recognize that this is a *very* important topic and one that you probably don't know enough about.

Somebody in your organization needs to develop standards for every kind of documentation: what's needed, where it should be kept, who prepares it, who reviews it and when, and whether and when it should be destroyed. This is a thankless job, but an important one. If nobody else is willing to do it, you should think about volunteering. At the very least, get the beast of documentation tamed in your own section or department.

Then call your attorneys and ask them to come snoop around and make recommendations. It will be much cheaper if you've done the groundwork, so the attorneys simply have to double check your work. The importance of reviewing written documents with legal counsel cannot be overemphasized. This step can save a lot of grief. In addition, your lawyer can tell you the "magic" words to place on documents to make them privileged communication between attorney and client. Learn them and learn when to use them.

This legal review pays off when the dreaded phone call says, "Your clinic is being sued for $10,000,000. As of this moment, no one is to destroy any record, document or note, under penalty of law."

Some quick, specific advice. If there is only one place where you are willing to invest the resources to do proper documentation, make it in the patient records. Good advice on how to do this is so commonplace we need not cover it here.

If there are only two places where you are willing to invest the resources to do proper documentation, make them patient records and personnel files.

When it comes to documenting personnel problems, here are the rules:

- state only observable and verifiable facts regarding job-related behavior;

- tell the truth; and

- keep it simple.

Your goal is to document what the employee was supposed to do, what the employee *actually* did instead, what specific changes you told the employee to make to comply with job requirements, the date by which changes must be made and the consequences of not changing. That's all. No speculations as to employee motivation or character. No questioning of honesty. Just the facts. Let employees read what you've written. Get them to sign it, and give them a copy. If they dispute your version of the events, let them note that fact in their own handwriting, right there on the same memo or form. If an employee won't sign, ask another manager to witness your request for a signature. Then note the refusal, and ask the other manager to sign as witness.

Hard ball? Self protection.

Final thoughts

After a weekend of spring cleaning, have you ever thought about how *ironic* clean windows are? When your windows are absolutely, perfectly, spotlessly crystal clear, what happens? Guests admire the view out the window, or they comment on your nice draperies... but nobody notices the windows. Why not? Because *they can't see the windows* — the windows are entirely too clean to be seen. Instead of seeing the windows, people see *through* them.

Good documentation is like that. Documentation is a thankless job. Like clean windows, excellent documentation often goes unnoticed. Ironically, the better your documentation is, the more people seem to "see through it" to concentrate on the matter at hand, on the issues that are so flawlessly documented.

When your computer commits suicide one night, and you have a nice, safe, fresh, completely verified and properly-labeled full backup right there in the fireproof safe where it belongs, because somebody remembered to do it, because they were properly trained, *because the instructions were clearly documented* ... Well, when that happens, it's reasonable to say that someone's obsession with documentation saved the day. But the odds are pretty slim of hearing, "Gee, someone's obsession with documentation saved the day; let's find that person and give 'em a big fat bonus!" No, you don't hear that very often. That's thanklessness of documentation in full bloom; that's irony, hard at work, reaping what it sowed.

When the state's Most High Inquisitor calls with a complaint from a disgruntled former employee, you get to say confidently and graciously, "I'll be happy to meet with you, and of course we will cooperate with your investigation fully. I remember the case fairly well, and luckily we have a personnel file that's just brimming with tardy slips and dismissal warnings, all nicely dated and signed by the employee himself." When that happens, reward yourself. Take a minute and look out your office window — that absolutely, perfectly, spotlessly crystal clear window — and admire the view. On a clear day, you can see forever.

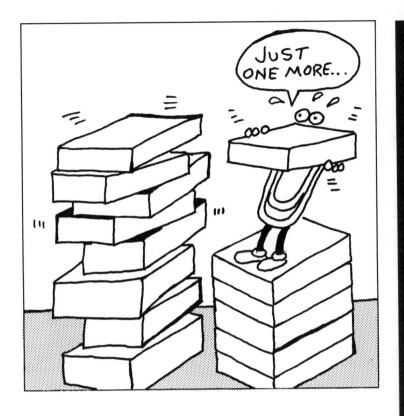

AXIOM

10

Know
when
you're
well-off

Every car owner should know a service manager like J.R. One of the authors took a car with transmission problems to him. J.R. said, "I can get it 90 percent right for about $150."

"But I want it 100 percent right. How much will that cost?"

J.R. replied, "You can spend another $500 to $800 and maybe get it 98 percent right, but it won't drive any better or any farther than it will at 90 percent right. That transmission is kind of funny. Ninety percent is about right for it."

J.R. knows how to achieve the best balance between investment and benefit when it comes to cars. Contrast that approach with the repair experience everyone dreads: You leave your car at a service center to have a light bulb replaced. Pick it up six hours later, and a smiling clerk says, "That will be $581.56, please."

"For a light bulb?"

"Well," she explains sweetly, "the technician said the alternator was not up to specs and probably caused the bulb to burn out, so he replaced the alternator and the drive belt and the idler pulley."

None of that with J.R. He would have said, "I noticed your alternator doesn't put out constant voltage. A lot of them are like that, but I've seen them run that way for years. Your lights may dim a little when you slow down, and weak bulbs will eventually blow because of it, but bulbs are cheap and alternators are expensive. I'll replace it if you want, but if it was my car I'd leave well enough alone."

J.R. not only services cars, he also sells used cars — with a 100 percent mechanical guarantee. He asks what kind of driving you need to do and sells you a car good enough to do it, unless you insist on buying one better than that. That's why the authors buy cars from him. Managers should develop as much insight into their operations as J.R. has with cars. Knowing how to balance investment with benefit is a valuable ability. "Light bulbs" costing $581.56 exist in medical settings, too.

This chapter describes "well-off," outlines methods for recognizing when your organization is well-off, and gives some reasons for leaving well enough alone.

These days, companies all over America are scrambling to train employees in the concepts of total quality management, or quality control, or continuous quality improvement. So is this book about to fly in the face of that movement by advising you to accept 90 per cent, when everyone else says go for 100 percent?

Not at all.

So how do you square the two theories? Let's let J.R. be our guide.

Whose yardstick is it, anyway?

The first question to answer when you are trying to decide whether your business (or some specific aspect of it) is "well-off" is to decide whose standards you are using. J.R. has different standards than you do. J.R. can feel the difference driving a car with an absolutely perfect transmission and one that's 10 percent worn. But very few customers can tell the difference. And if you can't tell the difference, what's the difference?

As much as $650, according to J.R.

J.R. is smart enough to know when to use his *customer's* standards, instead of his own, to gauge whether the car is performing well. In a medical organization, the best standards to use for some of the most important things are (surprise!) the *patients'* standards. Standards put forth by the doctors, other employees and managers, financial advisors, business partners such as HMOs, and regulatory agencies such as OSHA all are important, and have their place, and cannot be ignored. But patients are the best judge of the general quality of a medical organization: If your patients think you're doing a great job, you are "well-off" in some very important ways. If patients think you're doing a lousy job, you are not well-off in some important ways, no matter what your accountant says, no matter what the peer review board says, no matter what anyone else says.

Patients are experts at administering the "worth a dang" test. Managers need to know and use this technique. You do it by making an instant, global assessment of something. The only choices are "worth a dang" and "not worth a dang," and the judgment must be made without any further explanation, qualification, rationale, excuse or anything. Whatever you're evaluating is either black or it's white, it's good or it's bad, it's worth keeping or it ought to be trashed. That's the "worth a dang" test. It uses gut standards, and it can be applied with equal ease to people, equipment, software, departments or entire organizations.

Why do this? First, because it is exactly the way your patients evaluate you. And second, because it helps you know when you're well-off, which is the topic of this chapter.

This technique must be tempered in its use, of course. Let's say your laboratory flunks the "worth a dang" test. You can't just throw the lab in the scrap heap — you have to fix it. But in this chapter we're more interested is what's supposed to happen if the lab *passes* the test. If it passes, *don't fix it.* (You would be amazed at how many people violate this wonderfully sensible rule.) If the lab passes the test, it's "well enough" by the standards you've chosen to apply, so leave it alone. Don't fix it. Look elsewhere. Find something else to fix — something that *doesn't* pass the test.

And now to resolve the original conflict between CQI and "leaving well enough alone." It's easy. You do both. How? When everything about the place passes the "worth a dang" test, then you simply raise the standards. Raise them until something flunks the test, and then fix that thing: "That X-ray department was fine when we were a struggling little rural clinic. But the clinic as a whole has moved into the big leagues — and X-ray has stayed in the minors. For a first-rate clinic like we are, our X-ray department isn't worth a dang." That's how to make this work for you.

"For a first-rate clinic like we are ..." Those are the key words in the process. Those words define the standards. They tell whose yardstick you're using. "For a brand new car, this transmission is junk," J.R. might say; but he'd jump at the chance to put that very transmission in a ten-year-old car, because in that car it would be about right.

Passing the "worth a dang" test is one way to recognize that you're well-off. Another is the tuxedo test, which we will describe next as we continue developing the themes of recognizing when you are well-off and not fixing things that aren't broken.

The tuxedo test

The tuxedo is an amazing achievement in design: there's not a man alive who doesn't look good in one. This cannot be said of any other garment ever created — including the birthday suit. Men look good in tuxedos.

The tuxedo can legitimately be used as an example of a "classic" design. What that means is that the design *cannot be improved.* Every attempt to improve the tuxedo fails — although that doesn't stop people from trying. Wider lapels, narrower lapels, bigger shoulders, smaller shoulders, tapered trousers, tapered waists, odd fabrics and worst of all, colors! Nothing looks right when compared to the standard. A properly made tux from your parents' time is indistinguishable from one made this year.

It is immensely important for managers to recognize that there are things in life that cannot be made better. Anything that is truly a classic will be diminished by attempts to improve it. When something is at the pinnacle, it cannot go further up. It can stay at the top or it can slide down.

Now apply that thought to your organization, to its people and to the way it conducts business. Got any tuxedos there? You probably do.

How about that the payroll clerk who has never, ever made a mistake or missed a deadline? She qualifies. Don't try to improve her performance.

How about the mail room? The place looks like a tornado hit it, but they get the mail in and out of there *fast.* Leave it alone.

How about ol' Doc Able? He spends 17 minutes on every 15 minute appointment, getting "behinder and behinder" as the day goes on, but his patients never complain — because he gives them his undivided attention when he finally does see them. Dr. Able won't use the new dictating equipment, preferring instead to write detailed chart notes by hand. He takes patients' blood pressures himself, instead of having the assistant do it. He is demanding, but he is not unreasonable. He has never been sued, and while he is not the top revenue producer, he is not the bottom one either.

Leave him alone. What would you improve, his handwriting? Leave him alone. Leave the payroll clerk and the mail room alone, too. If you try to improve anything, you will foul it up. These things are better than "worth a dang," better than "well enough." They're classics. They're not subject to improvement, at least not on this go around. In the real world, it just doesn't get much better.

The best possible Arnold Burns

In that wonderful '60s movie *A Thousand Clowns*, the main character is an eccentric middle-aged man, Murray Burns, who doesn't fit in well with the workaday world. His brother Arnold doesn't have that problem; Arnold Burns is every bit as conventional as his brother Murray is odd. In one sparring scene between them, Murray claims that Arnold has made a life for himself that is dull, dull, dull. Murray says it doesn't have to be that way for Arnold. Arnold has talent and could be something unique, Murray says. Arnold ends the discussion by admitting that he is not perfect and perhaps not the best human being in the world. But still in all, he says, "I am the *best possible* Arnold Burns."

Arnold was saying you don't have to stand out from the crowd to be special. It's true, and it applies to organizations (like yours) as well as it does to people.

When everyone in the room is wearing a tuxedo, sure they all look alike: They all look great. Your department or your group practice or your clinic or your hospital doesn't have to be the best of its kind in the whole world in order to be worthwhile, special or valuable. Make your organization the best you know how to make it. Aim for and hit good, solid, achievable standards of performance.

Then go home and enjoy your life, and stop worrying about conquering the world.

We don't propose for an instant that you ever rest on your laurels, or stop raising the standards, or relax your efforts to improve things. We simply say that perfection is an unrealistic business goal. Efforts to achieve perfection can backfire if you are not careful, and will leave you worse off than you were before. That thought leads to the next topic, which is another reason to recognize when you are well- off, and to leave well enough alone.

Fixing it too well can break it

Everyone who "tinkers" at home or at work has broken something by fixing it too well. "The water finally quit leaking from this coupling, I'll jus-sss-st give it one more tweak." Ca-ra-aaa-ack! Drip, drip, drip! "We can get the fax machine on the desk if we move the computer jus-sss-st a bit more toward the end." Ca-ra-aaa-ash! Bzzt! Bzzt! Bzzt!

Dr. Godley's programming team developed a patient registration and scheduling system. They produced a quick-and-dirty, bare-bones program that did the minimum job. The appointment clerks loved it. It produced schedules for each day and each doctor. The program got confused by things like holidays and doctors' vacations, but the clerks knew how to make changes in pencil to the printed schedules and they didn't complain. They did not know the system was rudimentary, they just knew that it saved work.

Encouraged by the response to that program, the programmers set about doing it right. They developed a comprehensive, flexible and complicated program that did everything imaginable.

You guessed it. When the system went live, patient flow came to a halt. While the system did a lot of good things, it took too much time for employees to get what they needed *from* it and too much time to put what others needed *into* it. Standing alone it might have been a good system, but it broke the larger system — patient flow — that it was intended to support. The old system actually worked better.

As Jonathan's father said about his rusted-out, 25-year-old pickup truck, "It hauls what I need to haul as far as I need to haul it." An old truck that *runs* is better in nearly every important way than a new truck that won't start. The original scheduling system was better than what replaced it.

Don't interpret that to mean that new trucks and new software are to be avoided. Of course that's not the case. But a wise manager makes sure to see how the details fit within the big picture. Improving always involves change, but change doesn't necessarily involve improvement. Don't change things unless the change will bring about an improvement. If it won't, leave well enough alone.

Final thoughts

There is not an easy-to-define or easy-to-understand "bottom line" to recognizing when you are well-off. The way you judge things in this light is the old standby: by observation and analysis. You have to look at every part of your business, and then decide whether the effort to improve it is worth the cost (and the risk) involved.

For example, in most businesses a lot is done from habit. It is a good idea to regularly examine habitual behavior, and ask if the reasons *behind* the behavior have changed, even though the behavior itself has stayed the same. If that's the case, don't leave this alone; fix it.

A few years ago a medical entrepreneur thought up a great idea. He would establish a network of physicians who agreed to provide specific preventive services for fixed fees. He would then sell preventive medical care plans to consumers for fees higher than what he paid the doctors, thereby making a profit. He had been involved in medical insurance for years and from habit tried to apply for licensing from the agencies that regulated health care plans. But to his dismay he discovered no regulations to cover his novel idea. He was stymied, so he sought the advice of one of the authors, hoping to lobby for legislation to permit the creation of his network.

The advice he received wasn't what he expected: "Just start the business. There is no law against it." His habitual behavior had kept him from recognizing that he was well-off. A fresh look produced near magic results.

Again, don't use "Know when you are well off" as a reason to accept shoddy or inferior work. But remember that the balance between effort and results is important. Every human activity is subject to the law of diminishing returns, so the trick is to get acceptable results with an acceptable amount of effort. Just asking the question "What do we have to invest to get the minimum acceptable result?" will help you master the knack of leaving well enough alone.

Think of every problem and project as a headache. What is the appropriate treatment? Habitually prescribing two aspirin can be fatal for patients whose headaches come from a brain tumor. Lifting the cranium and peeking in is not necessary for a hangover. Most headaches require aspirin, brain surgery or something in between. Some headaches require nothing; all you can do is fold you arms and wait. A good manager finds out as much as possible about the administrative headaches and then treats the symptoms and the causes. What is the minimum acceptable result? What is the minimum investment required to produce it? The answers to these questions define the "well enough" to "leave alone."

J.R. learned to balance investments with results the way most managers learn it, the hard way. He fixed the wrong thing more than once, and he broke it by fixing it too well more than once. He is better at obtaining referrals than many physicians we know, and every "consult" he performs on a car teaches him more about how to balance investment with benefit. The results are happy customers and a thriving automotive service and sales business.

Some more final thoughts

As chapters go, this one is a short one. Know why? We decided to take our own advice and ... (you fill in the blank)!

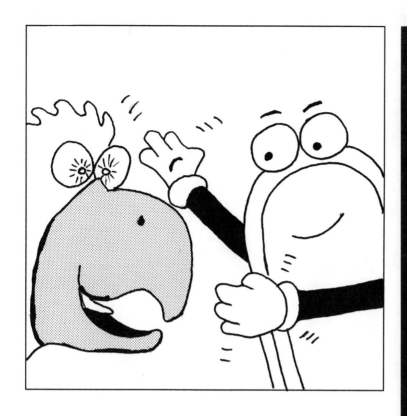

Quick, grab the parrot! Don't grab the parrot!

We began this book by saying that "effective management rests on a few fundamental ideas," and then we presented ten axioms that we consider to be fundamental ideas for management. We like to picture these axioms as items in a management survival kit. They are not a comprehensive theory of management, and they are especially not inviolable rules to apply in dealings with people. In the real world, theories and rules don't make things happen: people make things happen. Relationships make things happen.

We also said in the introduction that "how to get things done" would be the focus of this book. In conclusion, it seems clear that managers get things done through people. Managers who can form good and humane relationships with the other people in their work place have a much better chance of getting things done effectively than those managers who cannot.

So these axioms end up being about building effective working relationships. The axioms work even with people who do not want effective working relationships. Theories and rules come and go, but Dr. Godley will likely have tantrums until he retires. An effective working relationship with him requires insights and talents that don't come from rules and theories.

We wish we could say as a conclusion to this book that we put all the pieces together, they fit, and it's as simple as that. We can't, they don't and it isn't. Not only do the pieces not fit, pieces are missing even when it looks like they are all there. Management is not a neat, tidy, one-two-three process that follows fixed, clear rules.

Management is not exactly a craft, certainly not a science, and it is not art in the sense of museum art. It is more like street performance art. It can be structured or it can be improvised; sometimes there's a script to follow, sometimes everything is ad lib. Still, the show must go on; it's as simple as that.

Management is a lot like what happened when Nancy grabbed the parrot.

Nancy and her husband Tony were enjoying a late evening stroll around the neighborhood, when she saw something on the sidewalk in the distance, hopping toward them. What was it? They couldn't tell at first, in the soft light of dusk. It was just a vague form, about a foot tall, and it was hopping. Hopping rather oddly, actually. No, worse than that; hopping grotesquely. What was it? A newly evolved urban species? An injured puppy? Nancy's curiosity and urge to help sent her running toward it.

"Its a large parrot! Let's catch it," she said.

Tony yelled, "Don't grab the parrot!"

Too late. Armed with good intentions, she had cornered and grabbed the parrot. Armed with a beak that could crack ball bearings, the parrot returned the favor and grabbed Nancy's finger. And though she had gently grabbed the parrot around its body, the parrot had different motives: It buried the top point of its beak in the quick of her fingernail and the bottom point of its beak in the soft flesh below, and had every intention of bringing the two points together. Nancy's husband Tony is a scientist and he developed a theory about what happened next. In one sentence, here's the theory: Neural substances in parrot saliva and human blood make instant inter-species brain-to-brain contact, and one brain over-powers the other. The parrot's brain was obviously controlling Nancy's vocal chords, Tony thought; why else would such a torrent of raucous screechings and squawkings be pouring out of Nancy's mouth?

Nancy grabbed the parrot's neck with her free hand and twisted until the bird released her finger. She flung the thing down. It hurried away, unrepentant, degenerate and cranky, hopping faster and now even more grotesquely.

"NOW what are you doing?" Tony yelled as she ran after it again. She yelled back, "We have to catch the parrot. It could carry diseases! Help me!"

They trapped the parrot in a doorway. "Quick," she said, "Grab the parrot!" He did. It grabbed back, attempting to crack the ball bearings it apparently thought made human knuckles work. Tony immediately rejected his theory about inter-species brain-to-brain contact, and developed new theories about the relationship between pain and the rapid expansion of a certain type of vocabulary, and about the relationship between pain and a dramatic increase in the output power of the vocal cords.

Perhaps the parrot decided to turn loose because its mouth fell open in awe at the enormous number and range of familiar-sounding words, uttered with exquisite emphasis. Perhaps it decided to turn loose because Tony whacked it against a brick wall sharply enough to raise dust from both brick and bird. Who knows the workings of a cranky parrot's mind?

"Now, we really have to grab the parrot," Tony said. Again they cornered the bird, which had apparently developed its own theory on how it could make them go away. It used the 3-V theory: vocabulary, volume and vulgarity.

With not a whit of trans-species compassion, Nancy threw her jacket over the bird, tackling it and wrapping it into a tight muttering bundle. Now what? What does one do with a cranky parrot, whose pointed words and pointed beak add such emphasis to any point it wants to make? Tony squeezed the parrot into further submission while Nancy found a discarded cardboard box.

They boxed it, took it home, placed the first box in a larger and stronger box and left the parrot to ponder the error of its ways. They knew, and they hoped the parrot knew, that it might have a short career in the field of scientific research, should Nancy or Tony develop strange symptoms.

Their bleeding fingers looked worse, not better, after a thorough cleansing. How many millions of ambitious little microbes were now engaged in the pursuit of happiness in their torn flesh? Just where had this parrot been? What microscopic organisms considered the parrot's foul mouth a perfectly happy home until that wonderful stroke of luck that opened millions of even better habitats to them? Which of the infinite variety of urban sidewalk offerings had the parrot eaten? Had it gone back for seconds? With whom had it slept last night, and did it practice safe whatever parrots do?

Now imagine this scene, as Nancy and Tony imagined it. They go to the emergency room and join the typical Saturday night client mix at Urban Hospital. The victims of auto accidents are there, sitting next to some debaters who chose to express their positions with fists or other weapons. The debate team is sitting next to a group of imbibers and overindulgers. The imbibers and overindulgers are sitting ... Well, you get the picture. The staff is nearly overwhelmed. Someone finally asks why Nancy and Tony are there. They explain that first *she* grabbed the parrot, which imitated an aluminum can crusher on her knuckles, and then *he* grabbed the parrot, which again imitated a can crusher. And, they say, here's the parrot. Would the staff like to take it off their hands? Thank you very much.

They imagined the scene, did not like it, and decided to go to sleep instead of to the emergency room.

Managers must overcome challenges every day in order to take care of patients. Think of those challenges as parrot encounters. The only reason for managing relationships, processes, materials, meetings, discussions, projects and all the rest of it is to take care of patients. And when something gets out of whack, a parrot has you by the knuckle. Ask a simple question: How does this particular parrot help us do a better job of taking care of patients?

Management is the art of dealing with the parrot. Sometimes you are better off not grabbing the parrot at the time. Other times, you have no choice but to grab it. Sometimes, the parrot grabs you, and you can't seem to get rid of that sucker. Sometimes you grab the parrot in order to get it into a box and out of circulation. The task of management is deciding which parrot to grab, when to grab it, what to do after you grab it, and how to react when the parrot grabs you. But there is no choice about one thing: You must deal with every parrot that hops through the clinic.

The axioms in this book may help you deal with the parrots. The process is rarely neat and tidy. The axioms may give you a way of imposing some order and direction on chaos and uncertainty. Sometimes, though, things happen too fast, and you must tackle parrots and squeeze them into submission before you can even begin to think about axioms or anything else.

Every manager sometimes grabs the wrong parrot. Every manager gets grabbed by ill-tempered, nasty parrots. Every manager has to wonder about the consequences when parrots grab them. Every manager has to worry about how others will react to explanations of close encounters of the parrot kind. Dealing with all parrots, the nice ones and the nasty ones, comes with the territory.

In the real world, management centers on people, on human beings, with their enormous capacities for creativity and crankiness. People are not machines. Perhaps the greatest management mistake is unconsciously adopting the mechanical engineering approach to management. People are not like cars or phones or computers, with levers and buttons and knobs that reliably make things happen. Managers must plant and nurture and cultivate cooperative and productive *relationships with people.*

Is it radical to advise managers to acknowledge their own humanity and the humanity of the people they work with as a factor involved in getting the work done? Maybe. But it actually seems pretty logical to us. We're stuck with humanity until something better comes along, so it only makes sense to deal with it.

The authors have tried to give insights into managing effectively within that context. Dr. Godley, Jonathan, Ms. Short and the other characters portrayed all have real-life counterparts. We think their stories carry truths about management that elude theory and exposition. Getting things done effectively, compassionately, and in the context of humanity is one of the points of this book.

One manager complained bitterly to a consultant of the "stupid, incompetent people who work here." The consultant replied, "Okay. We've got stupid and incompetent people. That's as good a place to start as any. Let's work with it." The point is that whatever their strengths and shortcomings, these people were what the manager had. And the funny part is that a wholesale firing and restaffing would not necessarily improve the situation: we are often better off tinkering with what we have rather than replacing it. And we are certainly better off to roll up our sleeves and *do something*, instead of moaning about how terrible everything is.

We never get it exactly right as managers, in the sense of management as a process. But the *results* of an imperfect process can be superb, wonderful, perfect. It's like using the dysfunctional lawn mower described earlier, the one that was never really fixed and never really broken. We tinker, we adjust ... but whatever we do, we keep cutting grass. And when we're finished, the lawn looks terrific. It looks as good as it *can* look. It looks as good as it would have if we had used a brand new mower.

Here's a line we heard from a friend: Anybody off the street can run a business at a loss. Similarly, it is easier to make the lawn look nice with a new mower. We are tempted to say that anybody off the street can do it. Anybody can manage people who don't need managing. Anyone can get good work out of a team or a department of bright, industrious, hard-working and self-motivated people.

But what about getting the lawn to look nice using the mower we've got? What about the *do*-need-managing employees, and the team or department of *not*-exceptionally bright, industrious, hard-working, self-motivated, or-anything-else people? Who can get good results from them?

You can. *You can get terrific results from them.* C'mon, we're counting on you to figure out how to do it, and we just bet you can. It's hard work, but it's not that complicated. You can do it. But watch out for those green persimmons and those cranky parrots.

Robert Slaton, Ed.D., FACMGA, is Associate Vice President for Ambulatory Care for the University of Louisville School of Medicine, Louisville, Ky. Dr. Slaton earned his degree in Educational Administration from the University of Louisville and became a Fellow in the American College of Medical Group Administrators (FACMGA) in 1992. Dr. Slaton's many memberships to professional organizations include Medical Group Management Association (MGMA), Kentucky MGMA, MGMA Academic Practice Assembly, MGMA Multispecialty Group Executive Society, Kentucky Medical Association, American College of Health Care Executives and American Group Practice Association. Dr. Slaton is a frequent speaker and author on the subject of managing a medical group practice.

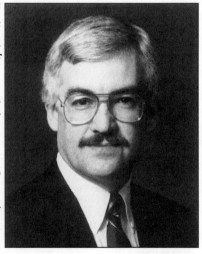

B ob Manning is Business Manager, Jefferson Internal Medicine Associates, a six-physician private practice in Louisville, Ky. Before joining that group, he was a marketing and software specialist for a custom programming house, and he taught computer courses at the University of Louisville. His earlier career includes positions as a general business consultant for a private firm, and many years work in management and marketing positions for not-for-profit and arts organizations. With a degree in English from Bellarmine College, Mr. Manning has wide experience writing and editing technical documentation for computer users, and he is the author of numerous marketing pieces for both print and electronic media. Privately, Mr. Manning is a script evalu-

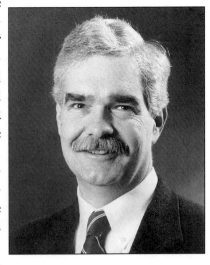

ator for a professional theater; he himself has written professionally for the stage, and was an assignment movie critic for *VCR Magazine*. Mr. Manning is an active member of the Medical Group Management Association (MGMA) and holds membership in the Louisville MGMA and Kentucky state MGMA chapters as well.

C lyde W. Jackson is a Human Resources and Management Consultant in Louisville, Ky. Mr. Jackson earned a Bachelor's degree in Psychology from Ouachita Baptist University, Arkadelphia, Ark., and a Masters in Divinity from the Southern Baptist Theological Seminary in Louisville, Ky., with additional study at the Univeristy of Iowa and the University of Louisville. His consulting practice includes helping dysfunctional organizations become effective, improving client service, implementing self-managed teams and assisting individual managers in improving their effectiveness. His clients include medical services management companies, long-term care facilities, academic institutions, retailing, food service, heavy 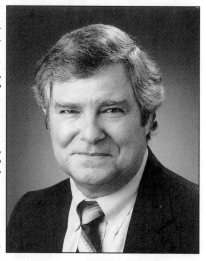 industry and manufacturing. Mr. Jackson's previous writings include two books, numerous business journal articles, and a weekly newspaper column. He is a featured speaker and seminar leader on topics relating to human relations, management and client service.